Claim Your Best Body

The Easier Way!

Six Concepts That Will Change Your Life

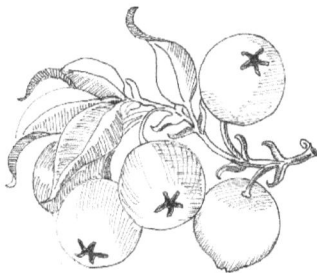

Sue Rose

ISBN 97809969829-3-1

ON THE COVER:

Sue's sitting on top of an organic, grass fed bison burger layered with organic, uncured bacon and embellished with fresh organic cheese, avocado, onions, lettuce, tomato, and watercress – *no bun.*

Table of Contents

Introduction

You want to know how to slim down (or stay lean), rid yourself of belly fat, feel better, lose the foggy brain, get more energetic, appear younger than your years, feel happy again, fix your health issues—in short, be your best self! But you don't want to spend your precious free time studying to be a nutrition and exercise expert. You don't want to go broke in this quest. And you don't want to fail.

This book is for people who want a simple, step-by-step guide that will show results. There are six chapters that correspond to six concepts you will learn – concepts that will change your life.

Claim Your Best Body is supposed to be easy-going. I'm trying not to give too much information for a good reason: I don't want you to be overwhelmed and frustrated. Still, I had to explain some concepts in more depth so that you would understand the *why* in order to be inspired to follow through with the *how.* If you get to feeling that "it's just too much", take a deep breath and relax. Let yourself coast for a while …and then come back when it feels better!

You may think I'm kidding when I say to take a deep breath, but I'm not. We've forgotten to breathe. Our breath is an amazing built-in de-stressing mechanism and we can use it whenever we feel that tightening up of our guts, or that overwhelmed feeling, or just free-floating anxiety. If we close our eyes and take a deep one, we can get back to ourselves, and things just get better.

After each chapter you will find a brief resource list that you can pull from if you really want to delve deeper into what's underneath my suggestions. I highly recommend you do that, as soon as you have the time!

All that's required of you is this: master the steps in Chapter 1 before you "break the seal" on Chapter 2. If you already know some of the steps in Chapter 1, that's great. You'll be on to Chapter 2 faster. BUT DON'T EVEN THINK OF GOING THERE until you have scoured the pages of Chapter 1—maybe even memorized them—and implemented each step in its entirety. Once you have mastered every step in Chapter 1—and that means you've assimilated all of the steps into your everyday lifestyle and you feel comfortable making those changes permanent…then you are ready to move on to Chapter 2; and so on, throughout this book. *Note: It doesn't matter how long it takes. Just keep making progress at your own pace.*

Consider this book your primer. I have attempted to sort through the growing body of information that's available and prioritize it, offering you the greatest benefit for your time, attention, effort, and money. The most important, yet fundamental, information comes first—to give your body the biggest boost up front. Each step, each chapter, and each sequential book will build upon what you've learned and continue to refine what you're doing as you move through them.

So, who am I to give you this advice?

Since the age of 16, nutrition and wellness have been my passion. I spent my adult life learning about healthy foods, movement therapies, east-west medicine, life extension, yoga, homeopathy, herbal medicine, macrobiotics, body-mind centering, cranio-sacral therapy, Ayurvedic medicine, hyperbaric oxygen, and every diet in the media. I was very physically active and took really good care of my body. In fact, my health and that of my loved ones always has been my first priority. Even so, by the time I reached the age of 47, I was a train wreck. We had been under severe stress for years due to our son's illness and death. I was cold, mildly overweight, and depressed. My optimistic outlook had all but vanished and I had a persistent haze in my head. I didn't feel good in any of my clothes. I couldn't tuck anything in or wear belts because of my belly. Life just felt like drudgery.

Something had to change. I began to research the new docs out there who were doing something called "anti-aging" and "preventive" medicine. A friend handed Suzanne Somers' book to me. After reading that, I researched and read about bio-identical hormone replacement. I wasn't going to accept one actress's assessment; I read Christine Northrop, MD, Dr. John R. Lee and more. I finally found a medical doctor/nutritionist team in the Chicago area (we'll call them "Dr. Longevity") who seemed a good fit.

For the next four years we spent upwards of $10,000 a year, and I dragged my husband 3 ½ hours each way, to our quarterly appointments with Dr. Longevity. I became their best and worst patient; I did everything they told me to, and the results were swift and complete. But I also asked many more questions than time allowed and my appointments tended to go on for twice the allotted time (to Dr. Longevity's dismay). The four years we were in their care became an intensive education for me. Even though I had studied nutrition and natural health for some thirty years before then, I was learning concepts that put a new spin on everything I once knew.

This was just one chapter in my education about health and vitality I am still expanding upon 15 years later. At the age of 62, I feel better than I did in my twenties. No kidding! If I didn't have a mirror I would forget all about my age. *Note to self: destroy all mirrors!*

In the first three months on the longevity program I lost 30 pounds of fat (picture 30 blocks of lard or butter), gained 20 lbs. of muscle (a net loss on the scale of just 10 lbs.), and went down 4 dress sizes! I had been wearing elastic-waisted, baggy size 10's and in three months I was wearing size 2 jeans! That was fun—and it was quite an ego boost. But it wasn't nearly as impressive as how I felt. I was so full of energy I could hardly keep my feet on the ground!

My girlfriends were all over it. "What did you do? How can I do it? I want to do it too! Teach me, teach me, teach me how!"

And so I did. Well, I tried. I started having cooking classes at my house and spent hours with my friends writing out equations and trying to teach them how to do what I had done. But it wasn't working for them – something was missing the mark. The strictness, the going without, the intense planning—these were challenging for anyone, and impossible for many. There just *had* to be an easier path to vibrant health. I was puzzled. What was it that prevented people from changing, even when they *wanted* to?

I had found my mission. I decided to find a way to make this easier to do, and accessible to everyone with an interest. I spent the next several years studying and earning my certification as a Nutritional Counselor. I began consulting clients and, as long as they continued to come for their weekly appointments, they were successful.

* * *

Here is a client testimonial from my nutrition practice:

"When I started working with Sue, I was experiencing periods in the day when I would get shaky and weak; it was beginning to scare me. I was also dealing with depression and general lack of energy. When I got to the point of considering medication, I decided it would be worth trying natural means before diving into the world of medications and their associated side effects.

"Sue immediately told me she thought I needed to stabilize my blood sugar and gave me a few dietary suggestions that I could handle. (I don't easily make changes to my diet.) I let her know that I wasn't willing to change my whole diet, so she suggested just a few changes that seemed "doable" to me and asked me if I would agree to stick to them for just one week. That was something I could handle.

"I was amazed how much better I felt the first day, and the improvements continued as days went on. I took Sue's suggestions for some supplements that made a big difference in the quality of my sleep and my mental outlook. My mood has lifted, my energy is much improved, and I'm able to work with enthusiasm again. Sue made it easy to understand, simple to follow, and she has done a great job of helping me to know what to expect next. Of course I have been singing her praises to my friends and co-workers when they ask me, "What happened to you?

"I've been following Sue's suggestions for four weeks now, and I am feeling so much better that I have no desire to go back to my old way of eating. Now, I'm getting ready for the next step. I'm counting on Sue to guide me with exercise and diet improvements that will give me even more energy and zest for life!"

F. C., Corporate Risk Manager

* * *

Several of my clients were obese, and dropped 30 pounds in about four months—at a very small fraction of the cost I had paid Dr. Longevity. But even at that bargain price, it was a catch 22: Who wants to spend their money to be told they have to change their beloved eating and lifestyle habits? Making a living as a nutrition and lifestyle trainer isn't easy. Ask any of them.

I began writing this book so that my clients would have a constant companion to refer to when they needed a nudge to get back on track—a simple guide that wouldn't require too much reading.

I decided to let the nutrition counseling business go and focus on my mainstay: public relations. The book sat half-written for three years, and then in September of 2014 I ran across it and re-read every page. I realized that I had forgotten some of my most important advice! I decided to follow the chapters in order, incorporating each step just as if I were learning this for the first time. Guess what? It works!

Do you want to feel great? Do you want to live a vibrant, full life until the day you die? Or would you rather decline slowly, through aches and pains and procedures and medications, and not-being-able-to-do-what-you-used-to-do, until you finally expire? It's your choice. I've chosen the former and I think by the fact you're reading this, you may be on the verge of doing so yourself.

It doesn't matter how late in the game you've chosen. Keep reminding yourself that your body's natural propensity is toward health and vitality. If not, you would have been dead long ago! Your body has an incredible impetus to thrive. All it needs is for you to stop mucking up the machinery—and all you need is the knowledge of what to do, how to do it, AND the desire to make some changes. Are you ready? Let's get to it then.

Acknowledgments

I want to express my sincere appreciation to Tony and Lizzie DiPaolo, my very Zen teachers, who taught me so much about life, acceptance, and pleasure. They have given me invaluable suggestions and inspiration for this book. To Daenah Rose, who has a way of breathing joy into everything, and to Barbara Miller—generous, lighthearted soul, for offering to edit my first draft and more. Finally, my eternal appreciation and love for my son Nicky, from whom I learned more than I wanted to about letting go and loving unconditionally.

Thank you.

Disclaimer

This book is not intended to treat, diagnose, or prescribe. The information contained herein is in no way to be considered a substitute for your own inner guidance and/or consultation with a duly licensed health care professional.

Forward

Prepare for Change; it is Useless to Resist.

Remember the Star Trek episode, "We are Borg?" Just as the Borg, change is also useless to resist.

Before you move into Chapter 1, I'd like to make a simple but relevant point: Change is not always easy. I'm trying to help make these changes easier, but let's face it—if you're reading this, the chances are pretty good that you've been consuming foods containing all sorts of sugars, sugar substitutes, and addictive chemicals—and you may have been doing it for a long time.

Doing some mental preparation will help. Because I've been eating real food for so long, the things I eat that taste plenty sweet with no sweeteners added may taste yucky to you at first.

I hope that you can look at the beginning of your program as a retraining of your taste buds.

The most difficult part of this program will likely be to have the patience and the willpower to give it a few weeks before unadulterated food begins to taste good to you! Please be patient with yourself. Don't expect to love the changes until you get accustomed to them. By then, you'll also be looking and feeling so much better, you'll be motivated to take on the next step.

Remember: *resistance is futile*...so go gradually and don't beat yourself up!

Chapter I:

Your Gut Brain (or "Why Am I In Such a Crappy Mood?")

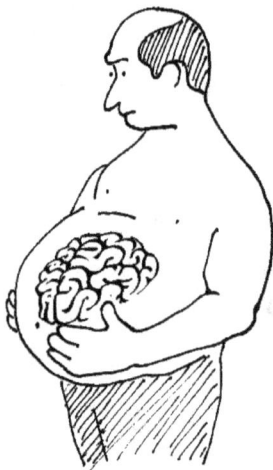

"YOU MEAN MY GUT HAS A BRAIN IN IT?

Maybe that's why it sticks out so much!"

* * *

You may have heard the term, "gut brain" and wondered whether it referred to your "gut feelings" or intuition. Yes, it does—but there's so much more! For a long time scientists and medical experts thought that the brain was the source of all information used by your body. But that's not the case.

According to Donna Gates, the expert on gut ecology, your brain and gut are having a constant conversation with each other. Out of the gazillions of messages that go back and forth between your gut and your brain, can you guess what percentage originates in the brain?

Only ten percent. The other ninety percent originates in the gut! Who would have thought?

How does this relate to your mental health? Guess where those wonderful neurotransmitters that put you in a good mood (e.g. gaba, dopamine, serotonin, epinephrine, and norepinephrine) are manufactured? You guessed it—in the gut.

If your gut is not in optimum health it's very likely you are not in the best of moods either. In fact, nearly every person I have worked with as a nutritionist has been depressed to some degree. And most people who are depressed find it difficult to get motivated to make changes that will lead to better health!

So which came first, the depression or the poorly functioning gut?

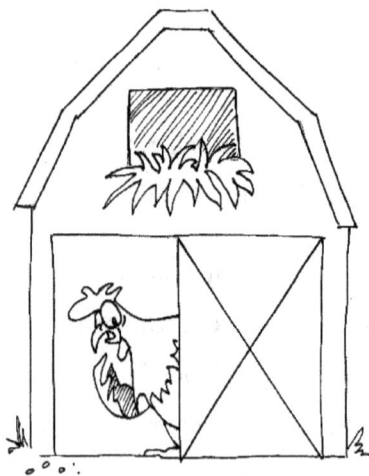

"Which came first – the chicken or the egg?"
we asked our 4-year old Lizzie. After some
thought, she retorted, "Well, the egg comes
from the chicken, and the chicken comes from
the barn." We thought, hummm. That's
certainly a new way of looking at it.

* * *

Sometimes a look at something from a different angle—even upside-down—can change your life. What if you stopped trying to lose weight or look younger or more attractive and improved your mental outlook first? Maybe the rest would just ease into place….

Your largest source of neurotransmitters is your gastrointestinal tract. Neurotransmitters are made from amino acids that must be obtained from protein in the diet. In addition to amino acids, vitamins and minerals eaten in food are required for the creation of the neurotransmitters. So you need to eat well, and that includes good protein sources, to get your "feel good" chemicals.

It follows that if your gut is deficient in microflora and impacted with gunk, you won't be able to absorb the nutrients that are responsible for making these neurotransmitters! And you are in a crappy mood. It's not your fault. Blame it on the food supply—or better yet—your dirty rotten knucklehead gut!

Your gut has been called your second brain. I can't overstate the importance of a healthy gut. The first step to your high vitality is to establish a healthy colonization of beneficial flora in your gut. This isn't only about improving your bowel movements, although that's a really nice perk! The benefits of cultivating a healthy balance of beneficial vs. pathogenic bacteria in the gut include (but are not limited to):

- Increased output of neurotransmitters that improve mental outlook

- Improved mineral absorption, which helps get rid of food cravings and makes you look and feel younger
- Improved thyroid function, which increases your metabolism (Gates asserts in her book, *The Body Ecology Diet,* that your thyroid function can improve by 20% with balanced gut flora.)
- Strengthened immune system
- Elimination of yeasts, fungi and parasites

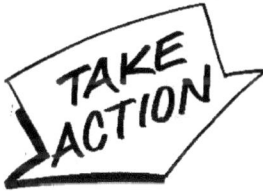

TAKE ACTION

1. ADD PROBIOTICS
2. CUT SUGAR
3. EAT CULTURED
4. FIBER UP
5. CLEAN COLON
6. UPDATE PANTRY

STEP 1: Load Up on Probiotics

NOTE: One jar of 180 capsules of Primal Defense Ultra will take you through the sequence I'm recommending in Step 1 below. It will cost you around $45. If you can't afford this supplement, read this step anyway, and then go directly to steps 2 and 3. You must do step 3 in lieu of step 1. But first, think about how much you're spending on the things that are mucking up your machinery, and consider a swap!

Junk Food Item	Price	Quantity per Month	Subtotal
Chips	$4.25	6	$26
Diet Coke 12pk	$4.99	4	$20
Fast Food Meal	$7.99	5	$40
Ice Cream Sundae	$4.75	4	$19

Bagel with Cream Cheese	$4.25	10	$42
Candy Bar	$1	12	$12
Pizza	$17.50	4	$70
Chinese Takeout	$25	3	$75
Total Monthly Outlay for Muck			**$303.50**

If this chart represents someone like you, we've just found a way to free up $303.50 per month to spend on whole, healthy foods and your probiotic!

Healthy people have a lot of good bacteria in their gut. This overrides the "bad" bacteria, which is always present. Many people today, however, have dysbiosis—an unhealthy balance of gut bacteria. This means the wrong kind is dominant.

When it comes to a healthy gut, HSOs are the bomb! Homeostatic soil organisms, such as those in Garden of Life's Primal Defense (no, they are not paying me), are your first stop on your shopping trip. These organisms eat away the crud that's impacted on your intestinal walls and embed themselves there so they can watchdog the place. They protect you from the ravages of the thieves, robbers and squatters that try to take over. They gobble up unhealthy bacteria, and allow the growth and proliferation of beneficial bacteria.

When I first went to Dr. Longevity, I asked him what he thought of the product, Primal Defense. (A healer had told me I really needed to take the stuff.) Dr. L., whose background was in biochemistry and lab research, said he had never seen an official study on the product, but that several of his patients told him they were using it and reported excellent results. That was good enough for me. I started using Primal Defense right then. Over the past several years, I have heard HSOs recommended over and over again by leading health experts. There are great benefits to loading up on these critters.

Primal Defense comes in a powder with a scoop, and in capsules. Since I'm all about making life easier for you, I recommend getting the capsules. Because you need both the HSOs (which are brown, like dirt) and a resident probiotic (resident probiotics are strains that you've probably heard of most often, like acidophilus, bifidus etc.), you can make this really simple by purchasing the Primal Defense ULTRA, which contains both HSOs and resident probiotics.

The Primal Defense ULTRA is *not* meant to be refrigerated, which makes this step really easy.

Keep the jar on your nightstand, next to a glass of water. (Get into the habit of always taking a large glass of water to bed with you.) Take one capsule right when you wake up. Follow it with a glass of water. Do this for one week. Then the second week, add one at bedtime. Stay at one in the morning and one at bedtime for a full week. Then increase to two in the morning when you wake. Stay there for a week. Then add a second capsule at night. Now you're at four caps daily.

(NOTE: Do not push this too fast! If anything, take MORE time to do this—not less. Your gut needs to adjust to its new residents. A family member of mine got overly enthusiastic and jumped right into several scoops at a time and got really constipated. Follow the schedule, please.)

Stay at 2 caps in the morning and two at bedtime for three weeks. Then start reducing your dosage by one capsule each week until you are down just one at bedtime.

If you have been making and consuming kefir, yogurt, and other cultured foods daily (step 3), you won't need the supplements anymore. If you won't do the kefir etc., stay on one capsule daily. If you are a man or a menopausal woman I don't recommend you take Primal Defense indefinitely because it contains ionic iron. Iron accumulates in the body unless you are either menstruating or donating blood regularly. (More on this in Chapter 6.) If this is the case, switch to another resident probiotic, such as Probiotic G.I. discussed in Chapter 6).

If you ever *must* take antibiotics or anti-fungal medications, you should start this all over again once you are off those medications. I was prescribed Diflucan (oral antifungal) once, and it messed my gut up for years. Be wary of killing off your gut flora. That said, there certainly *are* times when an antibiotic is necessary. Just remember to recolonize your gut by following the above sequence when you're done.

You get the most benefit from probiotics when you take them on an empty stomach. Some need refrigeration and others don't. The Primal Defense ULTRA is best *not* refrigerated (called shelf-stable), which makes it easy, because you can keep it with a glass of water by your bed.

Now that you've added probiotics to your daily regime, you're ready for the next step! But don't wait for months to do step 2—start as soon as you've purchased your first bottle of probiotics:

STEP 2: Stop eating sugar – or at least gradually cut down to a bare minimum.

Sugar feeds the criminals in your gut. Those bad guys—yeast, fungus and parasites—thrive on sugar. When you choose to eat it, eat dark colored, mineral-rich sources like black honey (go very easy), or grade B maple syrup (very easy on this too). Even white cane or beet sugar is better than high fructose corn syrup! Better yet, switch to stevia or lakanto—which are totally good for you. Stevia is easy to get, and

Lakanto is available from Body Ecology. Never, never, NEVER EAT ARTIFICIAL SWEETENERS. Examples of artificial sweeteners are aspartame, sucralose, malitol, and saccharine.

The differences among natural sugars

This is a confusing issue for most of us! It's best not to eat any sugar….but can you? Me neither. There are a couple of easy metrics I like to use when deciding which of the natural sugars to use – when I "occasionally" use them. One is the glycemic index, and the other is mineral content. Generally speaking, things that are darker contain more minerals. That's why dark honey is better than light colored honey. The glycemic index (GI) is the same on both light and dark, but hey—if you can get more minerals, why not? When looking at the GI, what you want to see is a low number. This index tells what kind of effect the sugar or starch has on your metabolism—notably, your insulin response. You'll learn more about this in Chapter 2.

Fructose, naturally found in fruits, turns out to be a really bad thing when it's not consumed in the whole fruit form with its naturally present fiber.

There's a reason I am recommending dark honey and not agave nectar. Agave nectar initially won lots of folks over because it has a lower glycemic index than both table sugar and honey. The pure science later showed that agave nectar is really not good for you, and has a tendency to convert to fat as well as encourage metabolic syndrome and Type 2 diabetes. The reason? It's made up mostly of fructose. If you want to learn the details, read this blog by Dr. Mehmet Oz: http://blog.doctoroz.com/dr-oz-blog/agave-why-we-were-wrong.

Stevia and lakanto (the only source for lakanto I know of is Body Ecology) each have a glycemic index of 0. That's perfect! The GI of xylitol is 7—still low, and xylitol is good for your teeth too. The GI on brown rice syrup is 25—not so bad. Raw honey is 30; maple syrup is 54; raw sugar is 65; high fructose corn syrup is 87; glucose and dextrose are both 100; and maltodextrin is 150.

This may come off as obsessive, and I'm sure it's not welcome news for many; but (OK, now is a good time to take that deep breath) I have to say it: Please don't even think about putting fake sugars in your body. They are vicious neurotoxins and they wreak havoc all over your body, starting with your brain. Many people who are overweight and can't lose weight no matter how little they eat, are victims of messed up metabolism, which originates in the brain, and is often caused by imitation sugars and other toxic food additives.

I feel apologetic when I say this because sugar is really hard for most people to give up. See if you can cut down gradually. Your taste buds will adjust. I have a sweet tooth that I satisfy with dark chocolate. It contains some sugar, but not very much. It's also not the fructose kind. And I buy good quality dark chocolate that is peppered with almonds (protein) and sea salt (balancing out the sweetness) and doesn't contain additives you'll find in the cheap stuff. One square is a perfect finish to lunch or dinner, and it satisfies my chocolate needs as well as my sweet tooth. Incidentally, I used to think I needed chocolate cakes and brownies, but what I was really craving was the chocolate—not the starch. Eating chocolate itself is definitely working better all the way around my waistline.

When buying packaged foods such as whey protein, be sure to read labels carefully. Avoid products that are sweetened with fake sugars. The only sweetener in a protein powder product should be stevia—never sucralose or other artificial sugars. And not sugar itself. If you're going to choose to eat sugar, put it into your mouth consciously! Don't consume it accidentally by purchasing products that contain sweeteners you aren't aware of. If you want to use protein powders, I recommend getting a high-quality one with no sweetener at all. Add your own sweetness with whole fruits and possibly a drop of stevia.

STEP 3: Eat cultured foods as often as you can, and at least once a day.

What are cultured foods? They are foods that are fermented and contain strains of bacteria and yeast that are helpful to your gut. Here are a few; some will sound familiar to you and others not:

- Kefir
- Yogurt
- Miso
- Natto
- Tempeh
- Tamari
- Sauerkraut (uncooked, with live cultures)
- Kimchi
- Fermented coconut water
- Kambucha, a tea-based fermented drink
- The wide variety of fermented beverages now available at natural food

stores. Some even contain chia or flax seeds for beneficial fiber and Omega-3 fatty acids.

What's so great about cultured foods?

Raw vs. Cooked

You may have heard about the raw foodies out there—especially some Hollywood types who are whatever percent raw. The benefit of eating raw food is that it contains enzymes. Cooking kills enzymes just as it does probiotics. Raw food, even meat, contains the enzymes you need to digest it fully—leaving no "ashes" in your body that can cause diseases such as arthritis. That's a BIG bonus.

However, some raw foods contain phytic acid and/or oxalic acid, which are anti-nutrients. Phytates and oxalates actually block mineral absorption. And mineralization is the name of the game! Minerals are your absolute best friends. Greens that are especially high in oxalic acid are spinach, beet tops, and chard. (Deep breath.) Raw cruciferous veggies like cabbage, broccoli, and kale, are high in phytates. Kale is high in both phytates and oxalates, so I simply won't eat it raw. Kale is definitely not a good candidate for your raw smoothie. Grains and nuts contain phytates, and I hate to admit it, but so do coffee and chocolate (my favorite crutches).

Does this mean you can't eat them? NO! But understanding how to mitigate the effects of the anti-nutrients in them will help steer you away from trouble. There are some benefits from eating these vegetables, so please don't become afraid of them.

Culturing solves the problem because the fermentation process breaks down the anti-nutrients. Baby greens contain less of the anti-nutrients than their grown-up leaves, and the acids in lemon, raw cider vinegar or balsamic vinegar help to mitigate the effects of anti-nutrients. You can also choose to take an appropriate enzyme when you eat them. With veggies high in oxalates or phytates, cooking removes some of the anti-nutrients.

If you want to eat raw and reap the benefits of enzymes while you absorb maximum minerals there is a perfect solution: CULTURING. Culturing destroys the anti-nutrients, while preserving the enzymes. Plus, a HUGE added benefit is that the culturing grows beneficial bacteria for your gut!

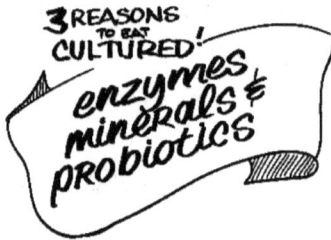

3 REASONS TO EAT CULTURED! enzymes, minerals & probiotics

Because grains and nuts contain phytates too, consider soaking or sprouting them. Fermentation works best; next best is sprouting; and then soaking. I don't eat much grain, but when I do, I try to remember to throw it in a jar and cover with water and a teaspoon of yogurt or kefir, and soak overnight. Then I rinse it well before cooking. Almonds taste amazing when you soak them. Sprouting is even better but more of a hassle for the time-challenged. Try soaking some in water for a day, then rinse, drain, and refrigerate in a covered container. Be sure to eat them before they grow mold. Yum!

Rather than freak out over this, remember that CULTURED/FERMENTED foods are GOOD. Use olive oil and balsamic or cider vinegar over salad greens, and when you make your raw food smoothie, choose veggies that are lower in phytates and oxalates, like carrots. Going back to the old adage: variety is not just the spice of life; it's also the healthiest! Don't eat the same things every day. Vary your greens and the way you prepare them, and you'll turn out just fine. See the resources section after this chapter for an illuminating chart that shows foods high in oxalates.

Sometimes Raw Is Not the Best Option

There are other reasons raw foods may not always be right for you. If you look into Ayurvedic medicine, you will find plenty of times that cooked food is better. If you do the Ayurvedic questionnaire at the end of this chapter, you will know your Ayurvedic constitution. If you are mostly Vata (like me), you can fly way off balance when you eat too much raw food without balancing it with the weight of liquid and fat. If you happen to be debilitated and/or anxious or are recovering from surgery, raw foods are not what you need at this time. See the Resources section after Chapter 1 to look into this further.

Yogurt and Kefir: How They Differ

Yogurt is not the only cultured food, and sugary yogurt is missing the point. Don't be fooled into thinking those packaged yogurts full of sugary fruit are good for you. When you purchase yogurt, get plain. Add your own fruit, in whole form. Try eating a half-cup of plain, full-fat, yogurt or kefir as a snack now and then. The full fat type tastes less sour than low fat. Dress it up once in a while with half a fresh pear, peach, or some berries and a few nuts on top for a treat.

True kefir is even better than yogurt! Kefir is made with kefir starter granules. These contain probiotics that are even more beneficial than those in yogurt. Unlike yogurt, kefir also contains a unique and very beneficial yeast organism. You can purchase kefir starter packets from Body Ecology by calling 866-423-3438 or going online to bodyecologydiet.com. They are also sometimes available at good health food stores. My Natural Grocers carries them. Keep the starter in your freezer.

Making Kefir is Simple

Making your own kefir is ridiculously simple. All you need is a quart-sized mason jar, milk, and kefir starter granules. To make a quart of kefir, heat up a quart of whole milk in a saucepan. Keep stirring the milk as it heats and don't bring it to a "skin" as you would with yogurt. Just heat it up to the point where a dribble feels almost hot on your wrist. Add your starter, pour into your mason jar, cover, shake or stir it up thoroughly (so you don't get lumps), and set on the kitchen counter for 18-24 hours. I like mine best at 24 hours. Shake your kefir and refrigerate. It will be slightly thickened but pourable; the longer it ferments, the thicker it can become.

When your jar is half-gone, take out 6 tablespoons of what's left and use that as your starter for your next quart. You'll be able to do 7 batches before you need to use the granules again. I always pull out the 6 tablespoons as soon as I notice I'm halfway down the jar, so that I don't accidentally end up eating it all and having to start over with the starter.

NOTE: Be sure all your utensils are sterilized. I run everything through dishwasher on the sanitizing settting before starting to make my fermented foods.

In the seasons when my home dips below 72 degrees, I wrap my kefir jar in a towel and put in an insulated cooler for the incubation period. This will keep it at a constant temperature for the fermentation process.

Why Is Kefir So Good For You?

Kefir contains 50 strains of probiotics, compared to about 7 to 10 found in yogurt. Kefir lays down a beneficial layer of mucus that these friendly bacteria can thrive in. It also predigests the protein in the milk so that it is easier to assimilate. People who are lactose intolerant can often digest kefir because the fermentation process actually digests 99% of the lactose contained in the milk.

The combination of calcium, magnesium and tryptophan in kefir acts as a sort of tranquilizer, helping to keep you calm and improve sleep. (I sleep better when I drink a "shot" of kefir at bedtime.) Your skin benefits too; kefir actually refines your pores over time. You can use it topically as a moisturizer and women can use it internally as a douche to implant friendly bacteria in the vagina, but this will happen automatically if you eat kefir regularly. There is good reason the word, "kefir" translates to "feel good" in Turkey.

I had a woman in my Meetup group who was excited to get started with Chapter 1, because she had always been rather willowy in build until she hit the age of 50, when she gained some weight and was feeling a slave to her cravings. She wanted her best body back. I promised her that tending to her gut health, plus a few tips from chapter 2 would nip those cravings in the bud. She emailed me the next day, and said that she couldn't find the kefir starter to make her own (which tastes really great on my palate) so she bought some ready-made, unsweetened kefir. She said it tasted awful and asked what she should do.

I suggested topping her kefir with blueberries and walnuts. Later I realized she had probably purchased low fat or nonfat kefir. When it comes to kefir and yogurt, choose full fat. It tastes much better—less sour. You can always add a drop of stevia for sweetness. Keep this in mind as you cut down on sugar. Stevia comes in powders and drops and is very, very sweet. Be sure to buy a brand that is made from the whole stevia leaf and does not contain maltodextrin or dextrose.

Miso, Natto, Tempeh, and Tamari: The Only Soy to Eat

I recommend people stay away from all soy products except for miso, tamari, tempeh and natto. Uncultured soy products like tofu, soymilk, and soy nuts, and, yes, even (darn-it) edamame, are fake food. Because they are not naturally fermented, they contain "anti-nutrients"— phytates, oxalates and goitrogens – which prevent you from absorbing the nutrients you need. The goitrogens in soy actually attack the thyroid gland, which could be one good reason so many people suffer from hypothyroidism today. (I'm one of them! I used to drink soymilk and eat tofu every day…and now I have to take a thyroid hormone. AGH! If only I had known then….) Of the soy food products, the only ones fit to put into your mouth are naturally fermented for two years or more. This natural fermentation process is the only way to get rid of the anti-nutrients in soy.

Tamari is naturally fermented soy sauce. The chemicals in the kind of soy sauce you usually get in the grocery store and at restaurants include neurotoxins, excito-toxins, and anti-nutrients common in unfermented soy "foods". Plus, the fermentation process is not natural— they use chemicals to imitate natural fermentation. You can buy regular or wheat-free tamari at any health food store, and now even in a growing number of "regular" grocery stores.

Natto and tempeh are fermented soy foods that I personally would rather not look at, much less eat. I invite you to experiment on your own! Miso, the fermented soy paste, comes in several varieties and is fun to experiment with. You shouldn't actually cook it, because the heat will kill its beneficial organisms. Just boil your vegetables and ginger in water and add a small amount of their broth to a tablespoon or two of miso paste in a bowl, mashing and stirring to dissolve. Gradually add more broth until you get a bowl of soup. Then, spoon in your veggies.

Cultured Coconut Water

When you buy Body Ecology kefir granules you'll get the recipe for culturing coconut water. For ready-made, the true, pure, cultured coconut water kefir is wonderfully healing. You'll want to get the unadulterated young coconut water that is cultured—no other ingredients. It's pricey. It will be clear and fizzy, and tastes a little sour. It is true medicine for your gut, anytime you are sick, or just needing a good boost. Drink a shot or two daily until you feel better. Or go on forever, if you can afford it!

Cultured Vegetables: Sauerkraut That's Live

The grocery store sauerkraut that comes in a non-refrigerated jar or can has been cooked, and so has no beneficial organisms left. You can buy live refrigerated sauerkraut, and it's expensive by my standards. I make my own. Most people won't bother with this, but I encourage you to try it. You can culture not only cabbage, but also other veggies. I've done carrots, daikon radish, kale, and mixtures of these and really loved them. I can't wait to culture some beets and see how they taste. Because more people won't bother doing this, I'm saving the "how to" to the resources section after this chapter.

STEP 4: Fiber Up!

"Experts" say you need a minimum 14 grams of fiber a day. If you add up your fiber, the chances are pretty good you'll come out lacking. I struggled with this for a long time because I don't eat much grain at all, and I'm sensitive to gluten. I tried psyllium husks (the active ingredient in Metamucil) but my tummy really didn't like it.

These days, I'm adding two tablespoons of whole flax seed into my NutriBullet (high power blender which pulverizes everything, including the seeds) on the days I'm making a shake. Flax is not the only option; chia seeds are also very good. They vary slightly in composition and both are a wonderful addition to your diet. If you buy flax and chia seeds, buy the whole seeds in bulk for the best value. Keep them in the freezer and grind as you use them.

Here's another very effective fiber option and you'll think it sounds disgusting, but once you try it you'll be a believer. I learned this from a wonderful naturopathic doctor.

It's whole flax seed, soaked. I get bulk flax seed and keep it in my freezer, since the oils in flax are not stable. Every morning (when I'm not putting the seed into my shake) I scoop out 2 tablespoons (you can work up from 1 tablespoon gradually) into a large drinking glass and fill the glass with water. The seeds need to soak about three hours before you begin drinking them. Soaking turns the flax seeds and water into a slippery mucilage. When you drink it, you can't even tell the seeds are there. You're getting good soluble fiber as well as insoluble fiber, plus the added benefit of some Omega-3 fatty acids.

Sometime around mid-day, I stir up the seeds and gulp down about half of the glass-full. Then I chase it with a cup of plain water. I do this again later in the day. That's enough fiber for my day, plus I'm eating lots of veggies for more. This technique keeps my bowels moving smoother than ever before…and I'm smiling more too. I have found mid-morning and mid-afternoon perfect for taking my flax. That's when I'm starting to feel hungry and the flax satisfies any cravings I might have. Additionally, if I want to eat something "bad", doing so after taking the flax slows down the digestion of the starch or sugar and that's good for avoiding insulin resistance. (More on this later.)

IMPORTANT: When you start out, work with 1 tablespoon and graduate up until you are comfortable with 2 or 3.

Soluble vs. Insoluble Fiber

These two types of fiber serve different functions. Soluble fiber dissolves in water, making the slippery mucilage mentioned above. It helps lower LDL (bad) cholesterol, decreases your appetite, and helps slow digestion, which helps prevent insulin resistance. Sources include: oatmeal, oat cereal, lentils, apples, oranges, pears, oat bran, strawberries, nuts, flaxseeds, chia seeds, beans, dried peas, blueberries, psyllium, cucumbers, celery, and carrots.

Insoluble fiber does not dissolve in water. It is great for moving things through the bowels faster. Sources include: whole wheat, whole grains, wheat bran, corn bran, seeds, nuts, barley, couscous, brown rice, bulgur, zucchini, celery, broccoli, cabbage, onions, tomatoes, carrots, cucumbers, green beans, dark leafy vegetables, raisins, grapes, fruit, and root vegetable skins.

Flax and chia seeds contain both soluble and insoluble fiber. Remember to keep your seeds in the freezer. The oils in the seeds can get rancid quickly when not kept cold. If you have ground flax or chia seed that's not refrigerated, throw it away. The oils in the seeds get rancid more quickly after being ground, so buy them whole and grind as needed.

STEP 5: Cleanse Your Colon Periodically

Colonic irrigation is the most direct, and the strongest way to cleanse your colon. It's not always appropriate for everyone. Don't do this if you are nervous or debilitated. Find a good colon hydrotherapy practitioner in your area who uses reverse osmosis water for the procedure. Never let anyone put tap water in you. (You shouldn't drink it either). Shop around and read what people have to say about the therapist. You need to feel comfortable in there!

Caveat: Some folks have a constitution that is very yin and cannot tolerate colonics as well as people with stronger, more yang constitutions. You need to be aware of how much you can handle. Knowing your Ayurvedic constitution can be extremely helpful in keeping your body's unique balance. The three Ayurvedic biological doshas are Vata (air), Pitta (fire), and Kapha (water). Understanding your constitution will help you to choose foods and food preparation methods that will work best for you.

Take This Quiz to Learn Your Ayurvedic Dosha!

Add up your scores for each of the three doshas, and keep this for future reference. V= Vata, P=Pita, and K-Kapha. You will most likely be a combination of all three doshas; if you score way higher in one of the doshas, that's your Ayurvedic dosha. If you score pretty close on two of the doshas and the third is significantly lower, you are a combination dosha. And if all three are pretty balanced, you're tri-doshic.

BODY FRAME

V   Thin, and usually have been; can be unusually tall or short

P   Medium, well-proportioned frame

K   Tend to be ample in build

BUILD AS CHILD

V	Thin as a child
P	Medium build as a child
K	Plump or a little chunky as a child

BONE STRUCTURE

V	Light bones and/or prominent joints
P	Medium bone structure
K	Heavy bone structure

WEIGHT GAIN

V	Have a hard time gaining weight
P	Can gain or lose weight relatively easily, if you put your mind to it
K	Gain weight easily, have a hard time losing it

EYES

V   Small, active, dark eyes

P   Penetrating light green, gray or amber eyes

K   Large, attractive eyes with thick eyelashes

SKIN

V   Dry skin, chaps easily

P   Oily skin and hair

K   Thick skin, cool, well-lubricated

COMPLEXION

V   Dark complexion relative to the rest of your family, tan easily

P   Fair skin, sunburn easily relative to the rest of your family

K   Tan slowly but usually evenly, skin stays cooler longer than most

HAIR

V   Dark, rough, wiry or kinky hair

P   Fine, light, oily hair, blond, red or early gray

K   Thick wavy hair, a little oily, dark or light

CLIMATE

V   Prefer warm climate, sunshine, moisture

P   Prefer cool well-ventilated places

K   Any climate is fine, as long as it is not too humid

APPETITE

V   Variable appetite, can get very hungry, but may find your "eyes were bigger than your stomach"

P   Irritable if you miss a meal or can't eat when you are hungry; good appetite

K   Like to eat, fine appetite, but you can skip meals without physical problems if you have to (not that you like to)

BOWELS

V   Bowel movements can be irregular, hard, dry or constipated

P   Easy and regular bowel movements – if anything, soft, oily, loose stools at least once to twice a day

K   Regular daily bowel movements steady, thick, heavy

DIGESTION

V   Digestion sometimes good, sometimes not

P   Usually good digestion

K   Digestion fine, sometimes a little slow

ROUTINE

V   Dislike routine

P   Enjoy planning and like routine, especially if you create it

K   Work well with routine

LEADERSHIP

V   Creative thinker

P   Good initiator and leader

K   Good at keeping an organization or project running smoothly

ACTIVITY LEVEL

V   Like to stay physically active

P   Enjoy physical activities, especially competitive ones

K   Love leisurely activities most

EXERCISE

V   You feel more mentally relaxed when you're exercising

P   Exercise helps keep emotions from going out of control for you

K   Exercise keeps your weight down in a way diet alone won't

MIND

V   Change your mind easily

P   Have opinions and like to share them

K   Change opinions and ideas slowly

EMOTIONS

V   Tend toward fear or anxiety under stress

P   Tend toward anger, frustration or
        irritability under stress

K   Tend to avoid difficult situations

DREAMING

V   Often dream, but rarely remember your
        dreams

P   Relatively easy to remember your
        dreams, often dream in color

K   Generally only remember dreams if they
        are especially intense or significant

EXPRESSION

V   Changeable moods and ideas

P   Forceful about expressing your ideas
        and feelings

K   Steady, reliable, slow to change

FOOD PREFERENCES

V   Like to snack, nibble

P   Like high-protein foods like chicken,
        fish, eggs, beans

K   Love fatty foods, bread, starch

ILLNESS

V   If ill, nervous disorders or sharp pain
        more likely

P   If ill, fevers, rashes, inflammation more
     likely

K   If ill, excess fluid retention or mucus
     more likely

SLEEP

V   Light sleeper

P   Usually sleep well

K   Sound, heavy sleeper

MONEY

V   You think that money is there to be
     spent

P   You think money is best spent on
     special items or on purchases that will
     advance you

K   Moncy is casy to save for you

SEX

V   Sexual interest variable, fantasy life active

P   Ready sexual interest and drive

K   Steady sexual interest and drive

NAILS

V   Brittle nails

P   Flexible nails, but pretty strong

K   Strong, thick nails

PERSPIRATION

V   Cold hands and feet, little perspiration

P   Good circulation, perspire frequently

K   Moderate perspiration

PULSE

V   Thin, fast, variable pulse, hands cold

P   Strong full pulse, hands warm

K   Steady slow rhythmic pulse, hands cool

THIRST

V   Variable thirst

P   Usually thirsty

K   Rarely thirsty

TOTALS: **Vata**_____
               Pitta_____
               Kapha_____

If you score high on Vata, be very careful with colonics and other cleansing methods. Go easy. Pay close attention to how your body feels afterward. Keep warm and eat lots of warm, wet foods like soups and stews with butter, ghee or coconut oil to weigh them down.

If you score higher on the Kapha side, you can tolerate colonics more easily and may want to schedule them regularly. Pittas fall in between Vatas and Kaphas. They can tolerate colonics moderately.

Most people can tolerate one or two colonics well. However, if you are really debilitated, weak, anorexic, or suffer from acute anxiety or nervous disorders, stay away from colonics. Use a more gentle form of cleansing, like a gentle cleansing diet for a few weeks.

STEP 6: Update Your Pantry

Ditch These:

- Sugar (refined)
- Soy sauce (if not natural Tamari)
- Accent (flavor enhancer; it's just MSG)
- Sodas
- Fruit Juices (more on this in Chapter 2)
- Spices that contain MSG by any name (refer to list of names for MSG in Chapter 4)
- Anything you already know is junk food

Stock These:

- Primal Defense Ultra
- Stevia powder or drops made from the whole leaf (not containing maltodextrin, or dextrose; inulin is OK because it is fiber-based and also feeds the good gut-dwellers)
- Kefir granules and whole milk OR ready-made kefir (whole milk, plain, not sweetened)
- Whole flax or chia seeds

- Miso (try all kinds and see what your favorite will be)
- Tamari (wheat free is available)
- Live cultured sauerkraut
- Yogurt (unsweetened, plain, whole milk)
- Other cultured foods and drinks you want to try

- Quality dark chocolate for a treat – the darker the better
- Dark colored honey for very occasional use
- Grade B maple syrup for very occasional use
- Hard candy made with rice syrup for those emergencies when you just have to have a sweet treat

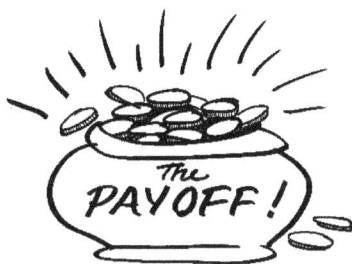

Now that you are taking probiotics, eating cultured foods, cutting way down on your sugar intake, consuming plenty of fiber, and cleaning up your colon, you should congratulate yourself! You're feeling better and becoming inspired to move forward to the next steps in your program. Your mood is better and your metabolism is humming along. You're absorbing lots more nutrients than you used to, so your skin looks and feels better. Your bowel movements are magnificent! Yay!

BUT WAIT! Take a pause and assess how you feel. Keep doing the steps. Get so comfortable with your new routine that it's second nature. Stay where you are until you are totally ready for Chapter 2. This could be months for you, or maybe just days.

Resources – Chapter 1

Cultured Food and Probiotics:

Gates, Donna. The Body Ecology Diet: Recovering your Health and Rebuilding Your Immunity. Carlsbad, NY. Hay House, 1996, 2010, 2011.

Rubin, Jordan S. The Maker's Diet. New York, NY. Penguin, 2004.

Oxalates in Produce *

	Vegetables	**Fruits**
Very Highest Oxalates (containing greater than 50 mg. per normal serving)	Okra Beets (greens and root) Spinach Swiss Chard	Fresh Tomatoes Figs (dried) Rhubarb

High Oxalates (containing greater than 10 mg. per normal serving)	Celery Collards Dandelion Escarole Kale Parsley Green Peppers Turnip Greens Watercress	Concord Grapes Kiwi

* *Best to culture or cook these, or eat them with vinegar or lemon juice.*

Kefir Starter Granules:

Buy from Natural Grocers or order directly from Body Ecology online:
http://www.bodyecology.com/digestive-health-kefir-starter.html. You can also purchase stevia and lakanto (natural sugar substitutes that are good for you) from Donna's website, along with a host of other good-for-you items.

Ayurvedic Medicine:

Frawley, David, O.M.D. Ayurvedic Healing. Salt Lake City, UT. Morson Publishing, 1989.

Morningstaar, Amadea and Desai, Urmila. The Ayurvedic Cookbook. Wilmot, WI. Lotus Light, 1991.

Making cultured veggies:

If you are not opposed to playing around in the kitchen on the weekend, I enthusiastically suggest you try culturing some veggies. I love doing this because it gives me a supply of perfect food on hand that requires absolutely no preparation! I need to just plan ahead every few weekends to chop and jar up some for fermentation. You can culture all kinds of veggies this way and mix them up.

NOTE: If your home dips below 72 degrees, you need to wrap the jars in a towel and put in an insulated cooler (yup—just like you do when fermenting kefir) for the fermentation process. It works beautifully.

1. Buy your veggies – organic cabbage, radishes (red and daikon), carrots—whatever you want to culture.

2. Buy Celtic gray sea salt or another high quality mineral salt (Himalayan pink etc.)

3. Get some organic seasonings if you like—I add caraway or dill seed to my cabbage.

4. Be sure to have good, non-chlorinated water on hand for the brine. Reverse osmosis or spring water are my choices.

5. Run all utensils through the sanitizing cycle of your dishwasher or run under boiling water. Shred up your cabbage or other veggies by hand or in a food processor. Put them in a big pot or bowl as you do this.

Reserve out a few leaves (cabbage or kale for example) to roll up and pack the top of the jar with. After all else is shredded, take a handful and put in the blender or food processor with some good water and about 2 tsp. sea salt and make a brine—which should be the consistency of medium-thick soup. Pack the veggies into your jar(s) and tamp down with a clean spoon. Try not to leave any air spaces. Fill with brine, (here's where you know if the brine is too thick…you want it to fill in all the spaces) leaving about an inch and a half of space at top of jar. Roll up a cabbage leaf or two coated in brine to fill that top space and cap the jar. Wrap in a towel and put in an insulated cooler for 3 to 7 days. Experiment to see how you like it best. With cabbage, I like 4 days best. When done, refrigerate and enjoy! When you've finished a jar of kraut, don't throw away the juice! Pour it over salads with oil instead of vinegar—you're getting those nice probiotics and it tastes great!

Chapter 2:

Become a Lean, Mean, Fat-burning Machine

One of the things we know today is that your health and longevity depend to a large extent upon your ability to burn fat efficiently. You really want to be a mean, lean, fat-burning machine. But why?

The immediate benefits of being in fat-burning mode are: When you are burning fat, you feel strong, energetic and grounded at the same time. When you are burning fat you are thinking clearly. When you are burning fat you are in your best mood. And when you are burning fat, you are not storing it! You are getting (or staying) lean!

The long-term benefits of being an efficient fat-burner are many. You will avoid the buildup of events inside your body that lead to biggest diseases of our day:

- Obesity
- Metabolic Syndrome
- Type 2 Diabetes
- Cardiovascular Disease, and
- Cancer!

By burning fat rather than storing it, you'll be stacking the vitality odds in your favor. So the first order of the day is, how do we put our bodies into fat-burning mode?

As a kid, my before school "good breakfast" was cereal, toast and juice. Usually I'd eat Captain Crunch, Sugar Crisp, or Cocoa Krispies, toast with grape jelly, and orange juice. Sound familiar? That was a "good breakfast" back in the 50's! Bless her heart, that's what my mom was told to do. And she was, and still is, a great mom. *But we know better now.* There is information at our disposal today that blows the old "good breakfast" paradigm right out of the water.

I'm going (yes, a tad apologetically—OK to take a deep breath here) to ask you NOT to eat cereal, NOT to eat toast, and NOT to drink juice for breakfast!

Bagels? No.
Oatmeal? No.
Morning glory muffin? Not.
Cold pizza? Nuh-uh.

Instead, I'm asking you to eat a *Killer* Breakfast.

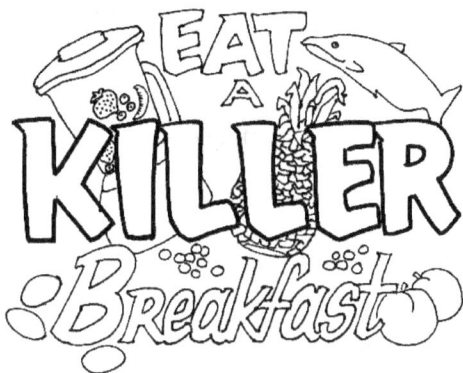

What will a Killer Breakfast do for you?

First, it's setting you up for a perfect, successful day. You will start your day in fat-burning mode. You'll feel terrific. You'll have lots of energy—but it's grounded energy, not the bouncing-off-the-walls kind. You're in your best mood and thinking clearly. And you won't need to grab a donut or the box of crackers or whatever's around the office mid-morning. In fact, you may forget about eating until it's well into lunchtime. (Oh, gee—it's 1:33 p.m. and I forgot to eat lunch. Guess I'll take a break....) All this you will feel right away—which is fun. But you'll also start stacking the odds in your favor when it comes to all manner of nasty health issues down the road.

Oh yeah-you'll be burning off your excess fat too.

* * *

A letter from a client:

"About 2 years ago, my "pre-diabetes" progressed into actual Type 2 diabetes. Since then, I gave up sugary drinks, including juices. I drank mostly water, black coffee or plain tea. In January of 2010, I just decided to go "cold turkey" on sweets. Since then, with an occasional relapse, I haven't had any cookies, cakes, candies, etc. I had a check-up in late January, and my A1C was 6.5. Since we were aiming for an A1C below 7.0, my doctor was pleased and cut my glyburide medication dosage in half, which normally should have raised it a few tenths from there. However, just six weeks

on Sue's "Killer Breakfast" brought my A1C down to 5.7.

Before attending Sue Rose's "Eat Your Way Younger in 3 Easy Steps" presentation at my company's headquarters in March, my typical breakfast was a large bagel— usually with avocado instead of cream cheese and sliced tomato. It added up to around 400 calories— 16 grams of (mostly good) fat, 12 grams of protein and 70 grams of mostly processed carbs.

Then I was fortunate to attend Sue's presentation at work. I had already been doing two of the three steps she presented, but I was intrigued and excited to try her "Killer Breakfast" and see if that would help with my blood levels next time around. I implemented Sue's Killer Breakfast right away. Other than the breakfast, and cutting my diabetes med in half, I really haven't changed my routine at all.

In early May, only six weeks after Sue's presentation, I had another checkup. This time, my A1C was down to 5.7. My doctor asked what I was doing. I told him about the Killer Breakfast I had incorporated into my daily routine. He approved, attributing my low blood sugar levels to that, and cut my diabetes med in half again.

We'll be following-up in August/September, and, if the numbers support it, he's looking to cut the med entirely."

- G.A., Corporate Finance Manager

* * *

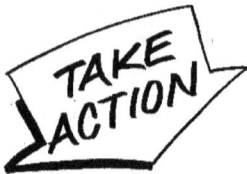

TAKE ACTION

1. KILLER BREAKFAST
2. EASE UP ON STARCH
3. PROTEIN SNACKS
4. WATER- NOT JUICE !

STEP 1: The Killer Breakfast

The Killer Breakfast is a perfect start to your day. Here's what's in it:

FOOD TYPE	GRAMS	EXAMPLES
Protein	24+	4 Eggs OR 4oz. Salmon OR 4 oz. Sausage OR Measured Whey, Egg white, or Vegetable Protein Powder; NEVER SOY
Carbs (non-starchy)	36-	2 Cups mixed berries, peaches, pineapple, pears, and veggies if you like
Fat	20-	1.5 Tablespoons coconut oil, butter, ghee, or olive oil; or a

		few nuts
Liquid	As you like	Water, Coffee, Tea, sweetened only with Stevia or Lakanto; but NOT JUICE

Note: You can eat more protein than 24grams. You can eat less than 36 grams of carbohydrate and less than 20 grams of fat. However, don't skip carbohydrates altogether; your brain needs them to function well! And don't go without fat either. Fat satisfies you!

Protein

First, you are going to eat 24 grams of protein for breakfast—OR MORE.

What does this look like? If you're eating salmon, that's about 4 oz., or a piece the size of a deck of cards. If you're having eggs it's 4. Sausage? 4 links. Or maybe two eggs and two links. If you're into smoothies, you're in luck because these days we have several choices of protein powders. There's whey, egg white, hemp, rice, (NEVER soy) and even raw protein from sprouted grains. Check labels to be sure you're only getting protein; if the powders contain carbs you'll need to figure that into your equation.

* * *

HINT: Take a look at the palm of your hand. If you were to trim off the fingers and thumb, you're looking at the portion size of meat you should eat three times a day (or equivalent protein from a non-meat source). Later you'll see that you also need some protein in-between your meals!

* * *

Carbohydrate

You have to balance the protein with the right amount of NON-STARCHY carbohydrate. This happens to be about 36 grams if you're consuming 24 grams of protein. Carbs= 1 ½ x Protein. If you're losing weight on purpose, don't go over 36 grams, even if you're eating more protein than listed in the chart.

For a Killer Breakfast, most people choose fruit for their non-starchy carbs because fruit's easy, it's juicy, and it's sweet. If you loosely fill a measuring cup with about 2 cups of berries, apples, peaches, pears or whatever you like (except for mangos and bananas, which are more starchy), you've got about 36 grams of non-starchy carbohydrate.

I'm the only person I know who regularly eats veggies (not potatoes) at breakfast. But with time and experimentation, you may want to join me! I love to make too many veggies for dinner, so that I can eat the leftovers the next morning with my killer breakfast—maybe in an omelet. Remember: potatoes are starchy, so reserve them for special times…they don't fit the killer breakfast.

I'm now using one of those amazing NutriBullet blenders. I put all sorts of veggies in it with some berries, fresh turmeric, bee pollen, flax seed, and a dash of sea salt. This is what I drink, along with two eggs scrambled in coconut oil. It's a perfectly KILLER Breakfast!

About leftovers: they're only worth eating the next day. After that, throw them out! Freeze them in portions when they're fresh-made to avoid wasting, rather than keeping them all in the frig and eating old, dead food.

If you're into food combining, the veggies mix better with protein than fruit does. But I have eaten a killer shake full of fruit and protein for years and it has worked just great for me. It's worked for many clients of mine as well. You'll need to experiment on yourself to see what works best for your body.

Fat

The ballast of the KILLER breakfast is fat. Fat is good. You need fat. In fact, if you know what kind of fat to eat, you can eat a lot of it! We'll get knee-deep into fat later on. For now, understand that if you're eating salmon you're getting awesome fat—the omega-3 fatty acid kind. If you're eating eggs you're getting plenty of fat and cholesterol, which is a GOOD thing (contrary to popular beliefs based on misinformation from the 60s—more in Chapter 5) in the yolks. And sausage—well, no worries. Plenty of fat there. The trick is to keep your fat consumption at or below 20 grams per meal.

The problem with animal fat is not the fat itself; it's the stuff that gets stored in it. All of those hormones, antibiotics and pesticides that mass-produced animals are given, plus the flight-orfight chemicals that the poor dears produce when handled inhumanely—all this junk gets stored in the fat.

If you can't eat all organic, you would do yourself a huge favor by making the commitment to eat organic, free-range and humanely processed meats. (I know. It's expensive.) The amounts of pesticides in produce don't even come close to what you ingest when you eat most of the meats that are mass-produced and sold in grocery stores.

At this moment in time, I can't afford the totally organic, humanely raised meats I used to buy. I do the best I can by purchasing the varieties that are not fed hormones and antibiotics. I also avoid meats that are injected with broth, which usually contains MSG and/or "natural flavors". It's worth noting that today in the U.S., federal regulations prohibit the use of hormones in the raising of pork and poultry! This applies to all pork and poultry—not just the ones that are labeled that way!

Antibiotics are another story. The label reading, "Raised Without Antibiotics" is important, because this in not a federal requirement. Animal health products not classified as antibiotics (such as some coccidiostats, which control protozoal parasites) may still be used. Yes, organic is best—but you've gotta have the cash.

What is organic meat? Here are a few of the key requirements for organic poultry, cattle and pigs:

- Must be raised organically on certified organic land
- Must be fed certified organic feed
- No antibiotics or added growth hormones are allowed
- Must have outdoor access

The animals' organic feed cannot contain animal by-products, antibiotics or genetically engineered grains and cannot be grown using persistent pesticides or chemical fertilizers.

The Good Fats

Cholesterol is something your body will make whether you eat it or not. Eating organic, free range, humanely raised and processed meats, eggs, and dairy products is incredibly good for most people.

The best fats for cooking are organic, unprocessed RAW coconut oil*, or organic ghee**. The best fats for eating raw are olive oil, organic raw coconut oil, and organic butter.

Avoid: PUFAs (polyunsaturated fatty acids), which are in vegetable oils. They oxidize and cause aging (such as atherosclerosis). They are also high in Omega-6 fatty acids, which we already tend to get a lot of in our diets. The balance can get thrown off when you ingest them in oils too. Again, we were mislead in the 60's and need to buck up and admit that we were blindfolded and led down a very dangerous path. (More on fats in chapter 5.)

*Coconut oil got a bad rap because of the kind they put in packaged foods, which is hydrogenated. Ick! Remember that the pure, raw kind is a great ally for your health and vitality. Just don't heat it so hot that it smokes.

**Ghee is just butter with the whey taken out, which makes it not burn like butter does. Both coconut oil and ghee are saturated fats, which (contrary to what we were taught for decades) are good because they are stable and don't oxidize easily. And they are very tasty too!

If you're one of the people who need to lose weight, you'll fall in love with coconut oil, which actually helps you burn stored fat! Watch how much fat you're eating for now (limit 60gm/day). Later, when you've reached your desired weight and BMI, you will be able to get away with eating lots more fat than you can now.

* * *

TIP: Always less fat than protein. Hard cheese; not soft cheese.

If you're trying to lose weight: When buying animal products like sausage and cheeses, you don't want a product that has less fat than protein per serving. Best to have less fat than protein. Equal fat to protein is OK now and then. So with things like sausage and cheese, when you are looking to them as protein sources, always look at the label. Most sausages will have more fat than protein per serving. Don't buy them. There are lots of chicken and turkey sausages available that have less fat than protein. I even found an Italian pork sausage (Polidori) that happens to have equal fat to protein per oz. Regular cheddar cheese has more fat than protein. Go for the low-fat varieties. Jarlsburg regular has more fat, but Jarlsburg Lite has less. Stay away from the soft fatty cheeses like Brie for now.

* * *

If you enjoy an easy breakfast that travels wherever you need to go, you're going to LOVE the Killer shake!

The Killer Shake:

- 1 to 2 cups whole fruit or fruit and veggies—not juice
- Water
- TBL organic coconut oil, OR handful of nuts to eat separately
- 24 g protein in protein powder (raw protein, whey, egg white, hemp seed etc. Never soy.)

Start with 1 to 2 cups fruit in the blender. (If you're using banana or mango, go light. Both are more on the starchy side. If you must, mix 1/3 banana or mango with other fruits that are not starchy.) Add water to cover slightly over the fruit (NOTE: Water, never juice). Then add your protein powder. You can choose from egg white, whey, rice, hemp or raw sprouted protein powders—but

NEVER SOY. If you like to add some yogurt or kefir, you can calculate the amount of carbohydrate in it and subtract that from the amount you're getting in your fruit and adjust the fruit accordingly. You don't want to go over 36grams of carb in your Killer Breakfast.

You'll also need to factor in the amount of fat in your yogurt. Don't go over 20 grams fat if you're trying to lose weight.

Some protein powder products contain fake sugars. Avoid them like the plague. Check labels! If you prefer a sweeter taste than the natural fruit produces, add a little stevia or lakanto, which are good for you. Watch out— stevia is incredibly sweet! I think it's better to learn to like things unsweetened. Your taste buds will adjust and you'll begin needing sweet stuff less often.

Read your labels. Measure however many scoops you need to get 24 grams of protein in your shake. Write down your recipe if it makes this easier to stick with.

Your shake can be personalized based on your knowledge and what you're working on. I usually add a teaspoon of local bee pollen, and sometimes some strong herbal infusions made from horsetail herb, pau d'arco and cat's claw in mine in place of the water (good green sources of calcium and powerful anti-fungal agents, as well as immune-boosters). The herbs make it taste horrible but I really don't care. (I'm accustomed to it. You probably *will* care.) I add fresh ginger, turmeric, and medicinal mushrooms sometimes. Some of my clients add maca and other superfoods. If you don't know about these things, don't get hung up on it. Go with the simple water, fruit, protein powder and fat recipe! You will grow your own recipe as time goes on.

Don't forget: Variety is the spice of life! Change it up! Vary your protein sources as well as your fruits and veggies. Experiment with herbs and superfoods if you like. Add things like cinnamon, ginger, Celtic gray sea salt—whatever you can think of that's good for you. By the way, a pinch of Celtic gray sea salt adds valuable minerals to your shake, AND makes it taste sweeter!

Pick the best fat you can to add to your killer breakfast. I alternate between putting in a big dollop of organic raw coconut oil, or if I'm in a chewing mood, I'll leave the fat out of my shake and grab a nice handful of walnuts to eat along with it.

Note on the raw coconut oil: It doesn't emulsify if your shake is cold. When you use it in your shake, start with about 1/4 cup hot water, add the coconut oil and blend well. Then, add your cold fruit, water, etc. and blend again. Otherwise, you'll get coconut oil lumps in your drink. A famous doctor you've seen on TV and online just adds a bunch of raw eggs for his fat and protein.

Recently, I upped my game. Rather than use protein powders I decided to go with whole, unprocessed protein. I now make my shake in my new NutriBullet blender with all organic ingredients. This thing is awesome. I start with a few handfuls of greens, then a carrot (unpeeled and broken up by hand), a stalk of celery, a chunk of fresh, unpeeled ginger, a chunk of fresh, unpeeled turmeric, a squeeze of lemon, two tablespoons whole flax seed, a grind of Celtic gray sea salt, a teaspoon of local bee pollen, a variety of berries or pineapple or pear, and some unsweetened cranberries –all with skins on. The NutriBullet pulverizes it all, including skins and seeds. I drink that with my two eggs, scrambled in coconut oil. Now, *that's* a Killer Breakfast!

In the winter I like to poach salmon and eat it for breakfast, either with last night's veggies, or sliced pears. You can devise all kinds of different Killer Breakfasts, depending on your preferences. Be creative, and spend a little time writing out recipes so that you have a guide—until it becomes second nature.

* * *

Let's drill down a bit deeper into the non-starchy idea, because it is the all-important switch that will turn on your personal FAT-BURNING FURNACE.

* * *

Low Carb vs. Low Starch

What is carbohydrate? Carbohydrates come from plant foods. They are long chains of glucose (simple sugar) molecules, linked together much like train cars. There are starchy carbohydrates like potatoes and grains, and there are non-starchy carbs like fruits and veggies. Non-starchy carbs are incredibly good for you. The problem with the "low carb diet" is that it doesn't distinguish between starchy and non-starchy carbs. The proper term would be "low starch" diet.

You need to eat all you can of the non-starchy veggies. Eat them until they come out of your ears and nose, really! Supersize your salads! Eat steamed veggies by the ton!

This is a very important distinction—starchy vs. non-starchy. It is key to your success in this program so please pay close attention to it.

One key difference between starchy and non-starchy carbs is in the links between their glucose molecules. Non-starchy carbs like green, yellow, red, and orange veggies and most fruits (not bananas!) have very strong, chain-like links. These take a long time to break apart. But the starchy carbs, which are mostly potatoes, grains, and anything made from grains and flours (any baked goods and pastas), have very weak, bow-like links. Bows come undone very easily.

Here's a simplification of what happens when you eat them:

Let's say you eat an apple on an empty stomach. Once you swallow the apple bites, they have to travel the length of your small intestines— around 25 feet—while your digestive juices work on those strong links to get them to break apart. One by one the links are dissolved and the glucose molecules trickle into your bloodstream – *gradually*. This is what you want. Your body requires that sugar to operate. But it doesn't want too much all at once.

Now let's just say you eat a piece of bread (read: starch) on an empty stomach. It's a whole different scenario.

The bread bites only travel two feet into your intestines before each of those bow-like links is undone. WHAM! All of the sudden the glucose molecules flood into your bloodstream at once. This is called a glucose shock. It's called a shock because it's not good!

In fact, you would die if all that sugar were to stay in your blood. Fortunately your body is equipped with a wonderful life-saving mechanism that takes care of you in the event you end up with too much sugar in your blood. It's called the insulin response. Your pancreas has the ability to secrete the hormone insulin into your bloodstream, which then tells those excess sugar molecules, "Get out of the blood! Get out of the blood! Store yourself in the tissues!" And, if you are not insulin-resistant, that's what happens. The excess sugar leaves your bloodstream and stores itself in your tissues as either glycogen or fat.

For simplicity's sake, I want you to remember the second storage option: FAT. Just think, "When I eat starch, I store fat. Eat starch, store fat. Eat starch, store fat." This should help you to remember why so many of us have a hard time losing weight, and especially that fat around the middle. We've been nourishing a love affair with starch all our lives! How many of us get all warm and fuzzy just thinking about warm homemade bread and butter? Chips and dip? Pizza, donuts, pasta, cakes, cookies and so on?

I have a secret to share with you here: FAT DOESN'T MAKE YOU FAT. STARCH MAKES YOU FAT. (Happy deep breath here.)

Remember when I said that your health and longevity depend on your ability to burn fat efficiently? Well how are you going to burn fat if you are constantly telling your body to store it?

The Sugar Connection

Sugar got blacklisted a long time ago. In fact, sugar not only sets off this insulin response, it also shuts off your immune system for hours after you eat it. Have you ever noticed that the people who are always popping candy and sugary drinks into their mouths are the same people who are forever catching colds? Those viruses are around all of us, all the time. Why is it that some people don't catch cold and other people are always sniffling? Sugar weakens your immune system for several reasons. It sets you up for dysbiosis (Remember chapter 1?) because those naughty yeasties and parasites thrive on it. There's more we won't go into here. But you know you need to cut down as much as possible. Go in increments. It helps to be gradual with changes like this.

Liquid Sugar is the Worst

When sugar comes in a liquid and you drink it on an empty stomach, it dumps directly into your blood stream. No intestinal transit required! What a rush! And what a glucose shock!! Congratulations…you just flooded your blood stream with insulin and successfully stored some fat! And that's not as good a deal as you once may have thought. By the way, even organic, unfiltered, unadulterated fruit juice is full of sugar. Fructose IS sugar and yes, it dumps into your bloodstream just the same as the sugar in Pepsi or Coke.

TODAY'S KILLER DISEASES BEGIN WITH INSULIN RESISTANCE!

Insulin was designed to be our friend. When we were Paleolithic people, we didn't have starches to eat. We were running around, spearing our meat, and foraging for shrubbery. Not much sugar around either…certainly no sugary drinks. Now and then on a really good day we might run across a berry patch.

If I were there, I'd gobble up every berry as fast as I could before the rest of the clan caught up with me! Selfish Paleo-Sue! And what would happen? All those berries with their natural sugars would cause a glucose shock and my pancreas might have pumped out a drop or two of insulin to keep my blood sugar in balance. Not a problem. Insulin was my friend. After all, it only happened once in a while…

But today haven't we changed our lifestyle a bit? We have maybe a bagel for breakfast, some wheat thins around 10am, and a piece of hard candy, then lunch is a plate of pasta and a brownie, then some chips and a root beer for a snack—and on and on.

Meal, after snack, after meal, day after day, week after month, after years…

We're telling our bodies to STORE FAT! Come to age 35 and look around you. Who doesn't have a little thickness in the middle? Maybe more than a little. Love handles and muffin tops. How many women over 40 are wearing belts around the waist anymore? And men—although they're wearing belts, they're ridin' low and it ain't pretty.

We've taken our old friend insulin and turned it into our ENEMY.

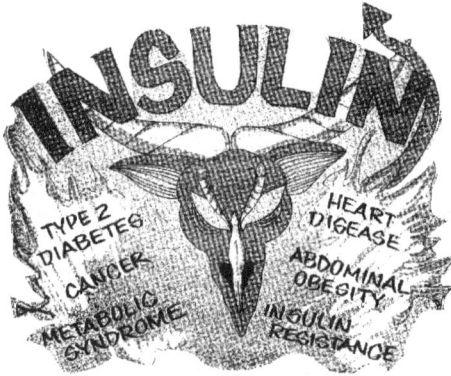

The very act of kicking off your insulin response sets you up for a cascade of events that lead to:

- Insulin resistance
- Abdominal obesity
- Metabolic syndrome
- Type 2 diabetes
- Heart disease, and
- Several forms of cancer!

Incidentally, pancreatic cancer is one of them. And doesn't it make sense? After all, the organ you're overworking for your whole life—the one that manufactures the insulin—is the pancreas.

* * *

There was a pow-wow in the fall of 2009. Some hefty non-government organizations (NGOs) got together and compared notes. They wanted to know what the heck was going on. "WHY IS IT", they asked, "that our world has gotten steadily more obese and sicker during the past 50 years?"

The result of that meeting was published in *Circulation, Journal of the American Heart Association*, November 10th 2009: Harmonizing the Metabolic Syndrome: A Joint Interim Statement of the International Diabetes Federation Task Force on Epidemiology and Prevention; National Heart, Lung, and Blood Institute; American Heart Association; World Heart Federation; International Atherosclerosis Society; and International Association for the Study of Obesity—a total of six NGOs.

They compared notes and what they found is that ALL ROADS LED TO INSULIN. At the root of obesity, Type 2 diabetes, and heart disease, is elevated blood insulin! This is big news. In another article published in *Cancer Prevention*, a national newsletter from New York Presbyterian Hospital, in the spring of 2005; Edward L. Giovannucci, M.D., ScD, Professor of Nutrition and Epidemiology at the Harvard School of Public Health, states:

"The link between insulin resistance and cancer may be related to the compensatory high levels of insulin….the higher circulating levels of insulin may have a cancer-promoting influence for at least some tissues. In the face of insulin resistance, some individuals may avoid diabetes; however, these individuals may be the ones most susceptible to cancer because they have the highest circulating insulin concentrations."

* * *

We've already discovered why our bellies get bigger as we age (read: Eat Starch, Store Fat). That's abdominal obesity, and it is linked to earlier death. What about insulin resistance?

Insulin Resistance

Consider two people with very different lifestyles. Betty is an active woman who doesn't eat much starch or sugar. She stays away from sweet drinks. Bill is a sedentary guy who loves to eat bagels, pasta, Snickers bars, any form of bread, and drinks soda daily. His favorite snack is thick-crusted pizza with a cherry Twizzlers chaser.

Because Betty rarely sets off her insulin response, her body responds differently to a glucose shock than Bill's does. Let's do an imaginary experiment:

It's Monday, 10 a.m. Betty and Bill are at the office and they both get hungry at around 9 a.m. Neither one has eaten breakfast. A coworker brings in a box of fresh donuts. Betty and Bill each eat a donut.

Betty and Bill both flood their bloodstreams with sugar and starch (the old 1-2 whammy) by eating the donut on an empty stomach. Betty's pancreas responds by excreting 3 squirts of insulin. She's fine. Unlike Betty, Bill has developed insulin resistance, due to his lifestyle of kicking off his insulin response frequently over the years. For the same incident (the donut), his pancreas has to excrete up to 6 or 7 times the amount of insulin as Betty's. So for the same donut, Bill has to flood his bloodstream with up to 21 squirts of insulin compared to Betty's 3.

Not only has Bill been packing on fat around his belly for years (eat starch, store fat)—he's also been developing problems within his blood vessels. That's because insulin is an irritant. It creates irritation in the blood vessel linings. After years of flooding his bloodstream with insulin Bill has developed tiny little holes in the endothelial linings of his blood vessels. Fortunately for Bill, his body knows how to patch up those holes—and it grabs some matter that's floating by in the blood, which includes cholesterol, and stuffs it up into those holes. That is the body's natural Band-Aid. And it's called plaque.

Bill knows he's got a big tummy but what he doesn't know (yet) is that he's been building up plaque because of his lifestyle all along. He wonders why his blood pressure keeps rising. He doesn't realize that as he continues to build plaque inside his blood vessels, there is less room for the blood to flow through and it pushes outward on the plaque-laden blood vessel walls. This shows up as high blood pressure.

It's not that we can't have a "treat" now and then. Betty won't have any lasting problem from that one donut and the corresponding insulin event. But Bill doesn't ever stop. He's eating sugary, starchy foods all the time, and drinking sugary drinks. He's ingesting who-knows-how-much extra added sugar, starch and quasi-foods in additives that are put into the fast food he's living on. Eventually his doc will probably have to tell him he's got something called Metabolic Syndrome.

Metabolic Syndrome: You're Almost Diabetic!

Metabolic syndrome is like a waiting room you get put into if you have three out of five of these symptoms:

- Insulin resistance
- Abdominal fat accumulation
- Elevated blood pressure
- High triglycerides
- Low HDL cholesterol (the good kind)

This room has two doors. You can pick either one. If you continue along the path you've been on, without changing your eating and exercise habits, you cross the room and walk through the door on the other side, which leads you to the Type 2 Diabetes room.

If, however, you choose not to go there, and you are willing to make some modifications to your lifestyle habits, you can turn around and exit the room altogether. You get to choose to avoid having Type 2 Diabetes! (And if you're already been diagnosed, you can actually get rid of it!)

All you have to do is follow the steps in this book. You can actually reverse some of your symptoms and become healthier than you ever imagined.

So just because of insulin, we've moved through abdominal obesity, insulin resistance, heart disease, and Type 2 diabetes. BUT WAIT— THERE'S MORE! At this date, six kinds of cancer have been linked to high circulating insulin: pancreatic, endometrial, breast, prostate, kidney, and colon. (Deep breath.)

NOW FOR THE GOOD NEWS:

There *is* a way you can turn off your insulin response and start burning fat all the time.

STEP 2: Ease up on starch!

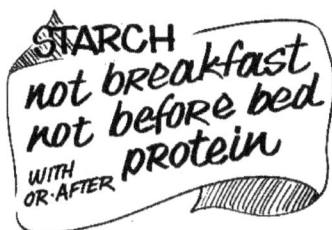

If you are eating a Killer Breakfast, you're starting your day burning fat. That's Step 1. Step 2 is: Don't eat starch (or sugar) before bed. I used to eat a huge bowl of plain popcorn before bed because I thought it was "free". It was natural, fairly unprocessed, and low-calorie. But every single time, I woke up with a hangover, even when I didn't have a drop of alcohol. I would feel fuzzyheaded, a little depressed, and sometime nauseous—and lacking energy.

Now that I know what I know, I totally get it. And believe me—I've experimented and it happens every time. If you want to wake up feeling fantastic, skip the sugar and starch and try having a protein snack before bed! You can even have a glass of wine if you want, or even two. But you need to have some protein (try low-fat hard cheeses, a handful of nuts, kefir with nuts, cottage cheese, hard boiled egg, meat or salmon jerky) to make this work amazingly well.

The second piece of this step is: Between breakfast and bedtime you have about 10 hours. That's when you can fudge a little. When you CHOOSE to eat starch (and sugar), always eat it AFTER protein! Think, "My first bite is always protein." A good rule of thumb is to eat desserts after a meal. How novel!

When you eat protein, you're probably getting some fat, and often some veggies, which contain fiber. Fat and fiber help prevent that big sugar dump by slowing things down. However, if you just decide to eat fat and fiber before your "treat" I fear you will not do well. Focus on tipping the scales toward protein and away from starch.

* * *

TIP: If you go out for Chinese food, do you order a huge bowl of rice with a dollop of stir-fry on top? No. Have a boatload of stir-fry and a little dollop of rice, or none. If you go to your favorite Italian restaurant for pasta one day, ask your waiter to bring the bread AFTER you get your entrée. Start with a nice portion of meat, fish, or seafood before you head into the noodles and bread.

And when you know it's a brownie day and there's no avoiding it, plan your brownie for after a meal containing a good amount of protein. It's that easy.

* * *

Ease up on starch means not for breakfast, not before bed, and always with or after protein. If you do this, you will burn fat.

And when you're burning fat, you are happier, thinking more clearly, full of energy, and not craving stuff. You may even find that you have to remind yourself to eat your next meal or snack.

STEP 3: Eat Protein Snacks!

This step applies to everyone, but is especially important if you need to turn your body composition around. If you have fat to lose, never go more than 3 or 3 ½ hours without eating. Back when I was transforming my body composition, I ate a hardboiled egg with half a fruit every morning at 10 am, every afternoon at about 3:30, and I always had some low-fat hard cheese with my glass of wine in the evening. Hey, more power to you if you don't drink alcohol! Just have a piece of cheese and, if you like, half an apple or pear—anything but banana or mango.

What happens with this is, you never allow yourself to get hungry, and you keep burning fat all the time. You will find that eating high protein snacks every 3 or so hours, you will lose your cravings for sugar and starchy foods.

Each snack you eat will have the same proportions as the killer breakfast only less— about half as much. So for me, a hardboiled egg and half an apple was a perfect snack. But I'm a small woman. For a big guy, a perfect snack might be two hard-boiled eggs and a whole apple. Or two turkey rollups (see below).

Zone and Balance bars are proportioned correctly—for me half is a snack, and a whole bar is a meal—BUT they are not made of real food. That's why I searched for food bars that are made without soy or wheat, are organic if possible, taste good, and have the right balance of protein-to fat-to-carbs.

Understand that most bars at the store are meant for marathon running and mountain climbing— they are not appropriate for a "going to work" day. They are high on sugars and starches and very low on protein. Although they are appropriate for mountaineering, you will get fat if you eat them otherwise. I've seen athletes get fat when they stop their training because they don't readjust their diets. When you buy a bar, look at the label. You want to see 22 grams or more protein and 33grams or less carbohydrate.

The Turkey Roll-Up

Another awesome snack I love to use in order to lose weight is some real (no injected broth and no hormones or antibiotics) sliced turkey inside a slice of low-fat Swiss for a "tortilla" and stuffed with julienne carrots and peppers and zucchini, or a dill pickle.

That's almost all protein! You can even follow that with some fruit. It is very satisfying. Use your creativity here—and you will be amazed how seldom you crave the wrong stuff.

STEP 4: Drink water, NOT JUICE!

I can't stress strongly enough that you must stop drinking sweet drinks. If you like fruit, eat it. When you put whole fruit into your smoothie, you're getting a limited amount of sugars, plus all the natural fiber present in the fruit, plus you're getting it with fat, and protein. When you drink fruit juices, you're dumping sugar into your blood stream—and if you think about it, how much juice would you get if you took your 2 cups of whole fruit and squeezed it? Not much. When you drink 8 oz. of fruit juice, you're getting a concentrated amount of fructose and kicking off that mean old insulin monster.

What to drink? How about water? Iced tea? Stevia is fine if you need it to be sweet. Herbal teas, iced or hot. Coffee. Have you ever noticed that really thin woman at the coffee shop who always pours huge amounts of half & half into her coffee? How does she get away with that? Well, it's the fat that's helping her stay thin. (Low fat diets suck, partly because you're hungry all the time, and partly because reduced-fat products often contain added starches to replace the fat that's removed.)

* * *

Tip: Buy stevia packets at the health food store. Then you can stash some in the glove compartment of your car, your purse, your briefcase, and your desk at work.

* * *

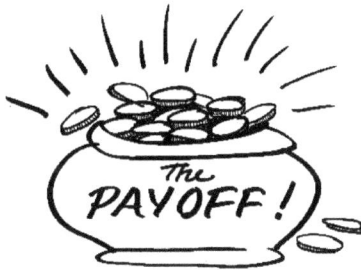

Now that you're

- Eating a Killer Breakfast
- Easing up on starch (not for breakfast, not before bed, and always with or after protein)
- Eating protein snacks between meals
- Drinking water instead of juice, and
- Forgoing artificial sweeteners

Don't be surprised if you feel more energy than you ever have before, your depression lessens or disappears completely- and you forget to crave sugary, starchy foods. Your blood sugar is stable. You are steering clear of diseases like

Type 2 Diabetes, heart, disease, and cancer. You feel more self-confident and smart—because you're thinking clearly again.

Have I mentioned you're losing weight?

Resources – Chapter 2

Thompson, Rob, M.D. The Glycemic Load Diet. McGraw-Hill, 2006.

Joint Interim Statement from *Circulation*

The Interplay of Insulin Metabolism and Athersclerosis from *Physicians Association for Cardiovascular Education (PACE)*

Insulin Resistance – a Lethal Link Between Metabolic Disease and Heart Attack from *Life Extension* Magazine

Insulin Resistance and Atherosclerosis from the *Journal of Clinical Investigation*

Chapter 3:

The Importance of Non-Exercise – OR –

How To Move Less and Burn More!

In Chapter 2, we learned how to use food to help our bodies burn fat. We focused on the insulin response and three steps to avoid insulin resistance and its associated diseases. Now, we're going to add a piece of the puzzle most people miss altogether—and it's easy, requires little investment, and pays dividends like you've never seen before.

Each of us has a different comfort level with exercise. In this chapter you will learn about several kinds of exercise – each with a specific purpose. Then, you get to choose what and how much you will do.

* * *

Paul Scott Mowrer once described my favorite walk, when he said, *"There is nothing like walking to get the feel of a country. A fine landscape is like a piece of music; it must be taken at the right tempo. Even a bicycle goes too fast."*

* * *

Don't Work So Hard, Sweetie!

Burning fat is easier than most people think. In fact, many people who decide to lose their extra fat get all excited about their new commitment and overdo it. When you work too hard, you can't burn fat! That's because fat requires a certain amount of oxygen in order to burn.

Let's talk about three heart-rate zones and what they mean to you. Whether you want to invest in a heart rate monitor or not, you need to understand this to get the most out of your non-workouts:

- Fat Burning Zone
- Fitness or Aerobic Zone
- Cardio Zone

In the fat burning zone, 80% of the calories you burn are fat calories and 20% are not. In the fitness zone, you're burning less fat. Only 30% of the calories you're burning are fat calories. In the cardio zone, you're not burning fat at all! Yes, you are working your heart muscle and improving your cardiovascular fitness and burning lots of calories, but you are not burning fat. That poor guy huffing and puffing and sweating bullets that you've seen on the treadmill day after day is working way too hard!

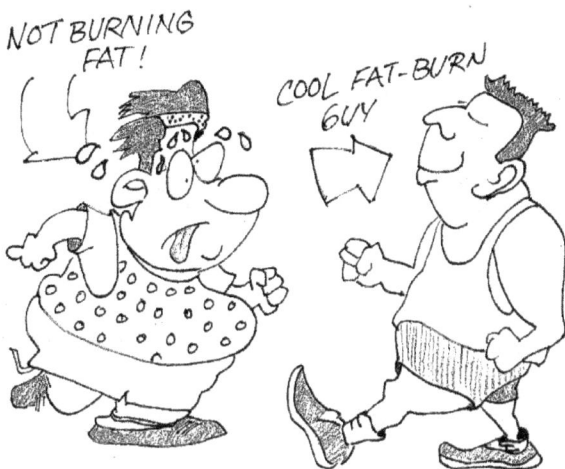

NOT BURNING FAT!

COOL FAT-BURN GUY

The coolest thing about this is that the fat burning zone is the EASIEST of the three. How do you know which zone you're in? That's where a heart rate monitor can be very useful. You can buy one for less than $150. But if you can't or don't want to do that, here's a good rule of thumb:

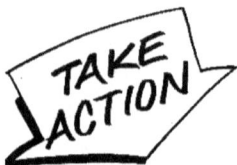

TAKE ACTION
1. FIND FAT-BURN ZONE.
2. WALK IN FAT-BURN ZONE
   5 DAYS A WEEK
3. SELF-PROPEL!

STEP 1: Find Your Fat-Burning Zone

Take a walk and …

- If you can sing the Star Spangled Banner, you're not working quite hard enough.
- If you can have a conversation, but not sing, you are probably burning fat,
- If you can't have a conversation, you are working too hard to burn fat!

Here's the easy way to calculate your three heart rate zones:

Heart Rate Zones

Max Heart Rate	Fat Burning Range	Aerobic Range	Cardio Range
MEN: 220 – age	Max x .5 to .7	Max x .7 - .8	Max x .8 - .9
WOMEN: 226 – age	Max x .5 to .7	Max x .7 - .8	Max x .8 - .9

If you want to know for sure that you are burning fat while you take your walks, get a heart rate monitor. Researchers found that it takes 20 to 30 minutes to activate insulin sensitivity.

Using your heart rate monitor, you will find that when you start out the door for your walk, you won't be in the fat burning zone right away. It takes a few minutes to get there, and at the end of your walk, it will take a few minutes to cool down. I recommend counting on a 40-minute walk to be sure you spend 20 or 30 minutes in the zone.

Insulin Sensitivity: KEEPING THE FAT OFF

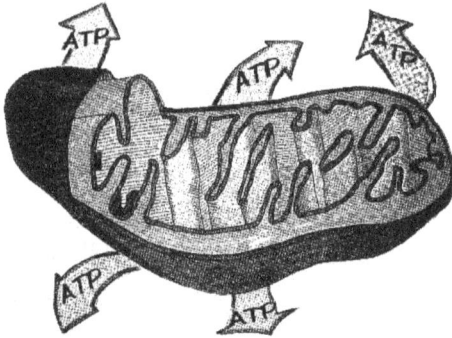

Can you guess what this little guy is?

It's a mitochondrion (not to be confused with a hypochondriac).

One makes energy, and the other makes excuses.

* * *

This is a little energy factory. There are millions of mitochondria in your body, and they are responsible for producing the simplest unit of energy that keeps your body alive: ATP. Interestingly, the mitochondria live in our muscle tissue. Most of them live in a certain kind of muscle called the slow twitch muscles. These are the large muscles that govern movement that requires oxygen, like your diaphragm and your larger leg muscles.

Remember what you learned about the insulin response? And remember that when you become resistant to insulin, you store more fat, along with all those other yucky things?

The mitochondria are where your insulin resistance or insulin sensitivity takes place. You *want* to be sensitive to insulin. That keeps you burning fat. When your body becomes resistant to insulin, you store fat.

The way you exercise can actually increase your sensitivity to insulin, thereby causing you to burn fat more often! It just so happens that your walking muscles comprise about 70% of your total muscle mass, and most of our mitochondria reside in our walking muscles! WHEN YOU USE YOUR SLOW TWITCH MUSCLES REGULARLY, YOU BECOME INSULIN-SENSITIVE, THEREBY BURNING MORE FAT, MORE OFTEN. Yay!

You've got three kinds of muscle fibers: slow twitch, fast twitch, and super-fast twitch.

Slow twitch fibers contract more slowly and require oxygen like when you are walking or jogging, and breathing (diaphragm). Fast twitch fibers contract quickly and don't require oxygen. You use your fast twitch muscles while weight lifting, and your super-fast twitch muscles are engaged in activities like sprinting.

Scientists did a study in Switzerland to find out which exercise worked better at increasing insulin sensitivity: walking up and riding down the mountain, OR riding up and walking down.

Results proved that riding up and walking downhill improved insulin sensitivity more. Hallelujah!

I don't want to discourage you from weight lifting or sprinting. But really, now. This book is about telling you the easy way to get to your body goals—and we're going step by step. Feel free to add in sprinting and weight lifting. But remember: When you exercise too vigorously, like the guy sweating on the treadmill, you go beyond fat-burn mode into fitness or even cardio, and you are not getting enough oxygen to burn fat efficiently.

STEP 2: Take a Fat-Burning Walk 5 Days a Week

If you have fat on your body you'd like to see disappear, walk in the fat-burning zone 30 minutes a day.

Do this 5 to 7 days a week to see quick results. If you are looking to stay lean (not lose more fat), you still need to do it, but only 3 days a week.

About Slow Twitch Sleep Mode and the Fidget Factor

Your slow twitch muscles will go into sleep mode unless you use them every 24-48 hours, depending on your normal activity level. People like me (hyperactive) who are always moving around, tend to stay leaner because they are keeping those mitochondria out of sleep mode. If you have a desk job, for example, you will need that walk every day. Fidgeters and people who move around at their jobs all day long may only need the walk every second day in order to keep the mitochondria awake.

STEP 3: Self-Propel

This is about doing daily tasks that add to your fitness, so you won't even know you're working out.

Park farther away every time. You'll be less likely to receive accidental dents in your car if you use the empty spaces at the back of the lot. And you'll burn more fat. Buy some 3 – 5 gallon jugs at the health food store and fill them up with reverse osmosis water. You'll also need one of those ceramic bases with the spigot. Carrying in your water jugs and turning them upside down each time you fill them gives you strength and balance training, and you are not loading landfills with needless water bottles. You're also not drinking tap water, which is not good for you! If you haven't already, try doing the yoga Sun Salutation for rejuvenation, balance, and stretching. This series of gentle movements stimulates your thyroid gland, which increases your metabolism, and tones your muscles too! Have you been taking the elevator at work and on your various appointments? Jog up and down the stairs instead! There's your cardio. Ride your bike on short errands instead of driving your car.

Self-propel. Every time, everywhere, choose the route that uses your body instead of a machine.

Stretch After Your Walk

My favorite way to stretch is to do the Sun Salutation. It stretches all or most of your muscle groups, stimulates the thyroid gland, and leaves you with a wonderful sense of wellbeing. Do it slowly, and hold each stretch for 3-4 seconds. Breathe.

You may find it helpful to watch this video of the Sun Salutation at https://www.youtube.com/watch?v=uMV4N q6jpu0 as you learn this flowing series of poses:

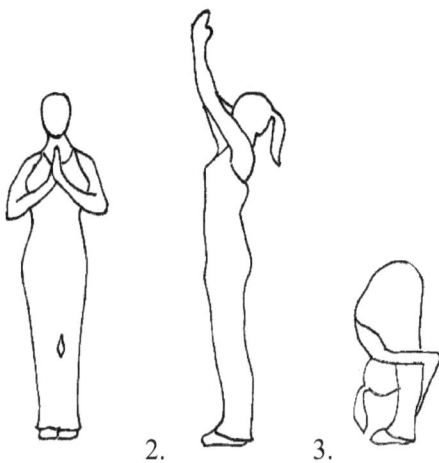

2.   3.

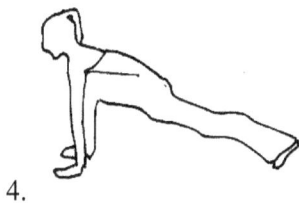

4.

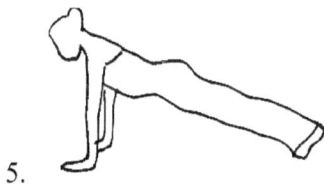

5.

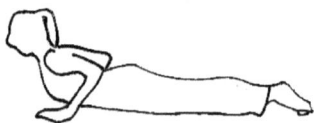

6.

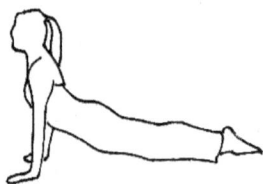

7.

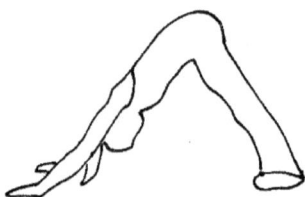

8.

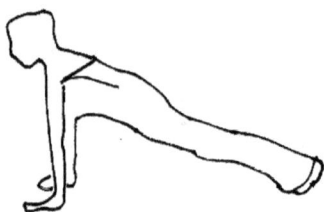

9.

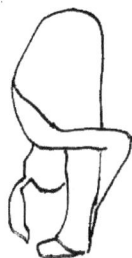

10.

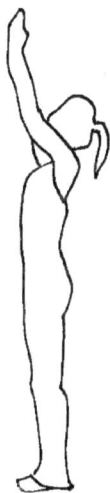

11.

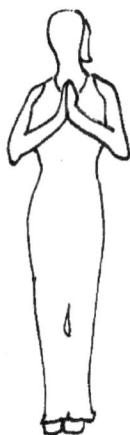

12.

More Traditional Stretching Exercises

If you don't like doing the Sun Salutation, or
like variety (like I do) try these stretches. Here is
a good 5-10 minute end-of-workout stretching
session:

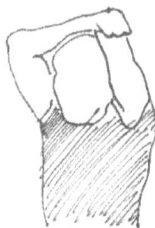

Triceps Stretch

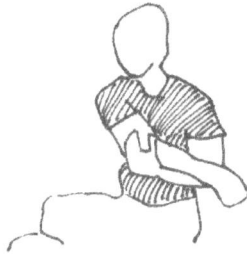

Shoulder Stretch

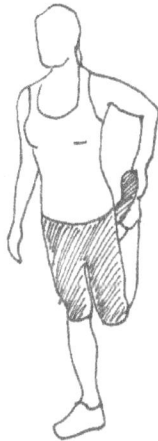

Quadricep Stretch

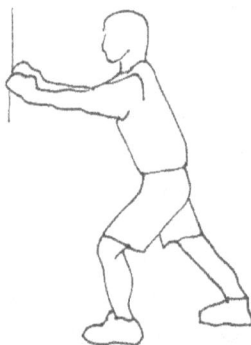

Calf Stretch

Hip Flexor Stretch

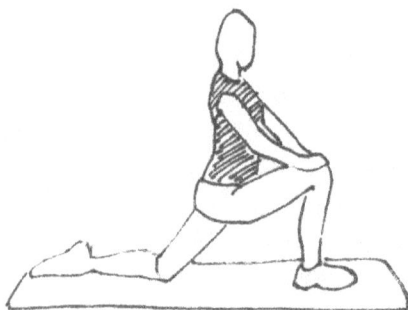

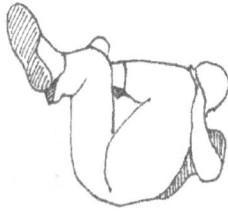

Hip/Glute Stretch

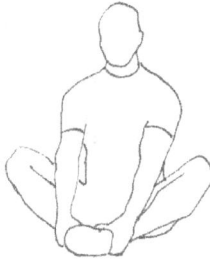

Butterfly Stretch

Hamstring Stretch

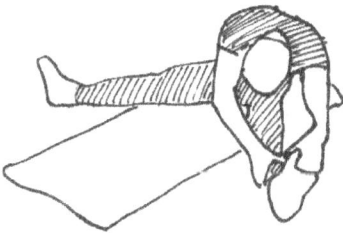

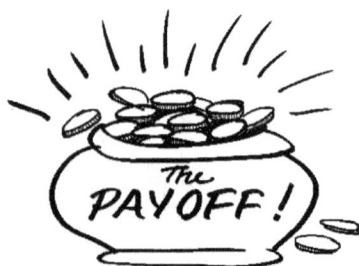

The PAYOFF!

Now that you've got your insulin sensitivity back on track, you are burning fat more often and passively— giving your blood vessels a much-needed break. You're also not overworking your pancreas. Getting or staying lean is getting easier and easier to do. You've learned that being gentler on yourself actually makes it easier to stay lean. Because you're stretching nearly every day, you're shaping your muscles, getting more toned, and noticing you're lookin' pretty darn good. You're moving more like a youngster too…all "flow-y" with those supple, flexible muscles!

PUTTING Chapters 1, 2, and 3 Together:

Since you're also taking great care of your gut brain (Chapter 1) and have turned yourself into a fat-burning machine (Chapter 2), I can't imagine anyone happier than you at this time. Take a moment to congratulate yourself! Enjoy your outdoor walks as well as those you do on a treadmill. Get accustomed to walking outside more often than not. Then, when you're ready, you can move on to Chapter 4.

Resources – Chapter 3

The Perfect Workout

I don't suggest going for perfection just yet. Go easy on adding new things to your regimen. However, if you're up to speed and just can't wait to add more, read on.

For those of you who have already mastered the fat burn and want to step up your game, you may choose to add to your workout. Strength training is fabulous, as long as you start small and build slowly. Increasing your strength means that you are also increasing your muscle mass. And when your body composition changes toward more muscularity, you will be burning more calories all the time. Muscle burns more calories. It also weighs more than fat; so don't worry if your weight doesn't decrease as fast now that you are adding muscle. I recommend not using a scale at all. Go by how your clothes are fitting and how you feel!

If you still want to add on to your workout, spend some time working a bit harder (fitness/aerobic zone) to increase your stamina and calorie output. Don't stop doing the fat-burn though—it's important if you are looking to melt away excess fat.

Finally, for those who want to go all the way, add some cardio training. It's going to make your heart stronger.

The Perfect Workout Includes All of These:

- Slow twitch walking in the fat burning zone
- Strength training
- Fitness/aerobic training
- Cardio Training
- Flexibility and balance training (Always stretch after, not before, your workout, when your muscles are already warm.

There's less chance of injuring yourself while stretching.)

Don't attempt perfection, though, unless you have moved step by step through these stages of fitness and it feels good to YOU. Jumping in too fast is a great way to burn out quickly.

Take it easy.

My favorite strength-building exercise: The Rotating Plank

You can find all sorts of strength exercises online, so I'm not going deeply into strength exercises. However, this one is just incredible so I'm including it! You can see a video of me doing this exercise on my website blog at, ClaimYourBestBody.com.

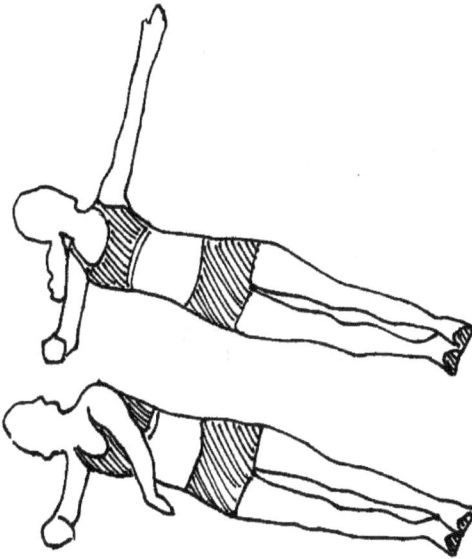

When you start doing this exercise, begin down on your forearm and don't use weights. Get your balance with your feet stacked and attempt to rotate down, looking through as you reach your hand underneath and rotate; then go back up with the arm. If it's too difficult to balance with your feet stacked, you can put one foot just in front of the other. Do three sets of ten repetitions on each side. Once you get stronger, move up onto your hand, so that your supporting arm is straight. This will be a challenge. Again, do three sets of ten on each side. When you are not struggling with this any more, try adding a light weight—say 2lbs. Build up on the weight, and if you're putting one foot in front of the other, see if you can get good at having your feet stacked. This is an amazing exercise for building core strength along with working your obliques, shoulders, triceps, and back. *Shapely, shapely, shapely!*

More on Heart Rate Calculations

The Karvonen Formula is a more accurate way to calculate your target heart rate, but it's more complicated than the simple method described in chapter 3. First, when you wake up in the morning, before you move around, get your resting heart rate. (Or rest for at least 30 minutes and then get it.)

Count how many beats in a minute. Then you can calculate your fat burning, aerobic, and cardio zones like this:

FAT BURNING HEART RATE (using R as resting heart rate)

$206.9 - (.67 \times age) = a$

$a - R = b$

$b \times .65 = c$

$c + R =$ fat burning heart rate.

AEROBIC/FITNESS RATE (using R as resting heart rate) $206.9 - (.67 \times age) = a$

$a - R = b$

$b \times .75 = c$

$c + R =$ aerobic heart rate.

CARDIO RATE (using R as resting heart rate)

$206.9 - (.67 \times age) = a$

a − R = b

b x .85 = c

c + R = cardio heart rate.

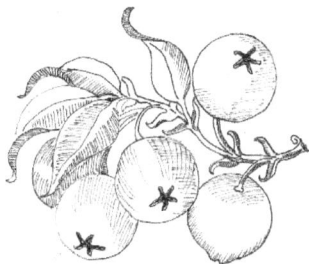

Chapter 4:

Eat Real Food

If you look at the movies Food Inc. and Food Matters and read The Whole Soy Story and Fast Food Nation, you are certain to gain a new perspective on the menu we've been served. However, rather than getting bogged down by it and becoming afraid of food, let's try to remember that each of us can choose to make better choices one choice at a time! Slow and steady.

* * *

In Fast Food Nation, Eric Schlosser writes, "A typical artificial strawberry flavor, like the kind found in a Burger King strawberry milk shake, contains the following 49 ingredients: amyl acetate, amyl butyrate, amyl valerate, anethol, anisyl formate, benzyl acetate, benzyl isobutyrate, butyric acid, cinnamyl isobutyrate, cinnamyl valerate, cognac essential oil, diacetyl, dipropyl ketone, ethyl acetate, ethyl amyl ketone, ethyl butyrate, ethyl cinnamate, ethyl heptanoate, ethyl heptylate, ethyl lactate, ethyl methylphenylglycidate, ethyl nitrate, ethyl propionate, ethyl valerate, heliotropin, hydroxyphenyl-2-butanone (10 percent solution in alcohol), a-ionone, isobutyl anthranilate, isobutyl butyrate, lemon essential oil, maltol, 4-methylacetophenone, methyl anthranilate, methyl benzoate, methyl cinnamate, methyl heptine carbonate, methyl naphthyl ketone, methyl salicylate, mint essential oil, neroli essential oil, nerolin, neryl isobutyrate, orris butter, phenethyl alcohol, rose, rum ether, g-undecalactone, vanillin, and solvent.

Solvent?

* * *

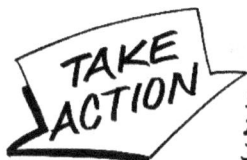

TAKE ACTION

1. READ LABELS
2. LIMIT FAST FOOD
3. FERMENTED SOY ONLY
4. COOK MORE OFTEN
5. PLAN AHEAD

STEP 1: Read Labels

The additives commonly used in what you think is hamburger meat, such as "texturized vegetable protein", are actually by-products of soy processing and contain neurotoxins. Just the single chemical, monosodium glutamate (MSG) goes by so many names it's hard for consumers to keep track of it. And that's just the point. One reason it's been slyly hidden in our processed foods is that it creates a craving for more foods containing the stuff. Following is a list of food additives that contain the highest percentages of MSG.

Names for MSG:

- MSG
- Monosodium glutamate
- Monopotassium glutamate
- Glutamic Acid
- Vegetable Protein Extract
- Gelatin
- Hydrolyzed Vegetable Protein (HVP)
- Hydrolyzed Plant Protein (HPP)
- Autolyzed Plant Protein
- Sodium Caseinate
- Senomyx
- Calcium Caseinate
- Textured Protein
- Yeast Extract
- Yeast food or nutrient
- Autolyzed Yeast

All of the above should be avoided! They mess up the neuroreceptors in your brain.

Natural Flavors – *What Are They?*

Don't make assumptions about products and storefronts that claim to be "healthy". (Deep breath.) I am astounded that I can go to my favorite health food stores and find yeast extract on many labels. I've become so aware of the "taste" of MSG and "natural flavors" that I can feel a cracker or chip fizzle on my tongue and I will immediately spit it out. Then, after a careful review of the ingredient label I'll usually find "yeast extract" or "natural flavors" listed.

Finding a clear answer on what "natural flavorings" actually are is confusing at best. What I've come to learn is that both "artificial" and "natural" flavorings are made in a laboratory by someone called a "flavorist". The reason this person has a job is that food manufacturers want to make their cheap, processed "foods" taste so irresistibly good that you'll keep coming back for more. They engineer very intense flavor sensations that quickly fade, so that you'll want to keep on eating, even though you're not hungry. You've just got to have more! The only difference between an artificial flavor and a "natural" flavor is that the original molecule used (in a "natural" flavoring) came from a natural food, say a piece of cheese. A molecule. Then it was engineered in a laboratory and changed into something chemically based and cheap so that the food manufacturer can make bland, stale, dead food taste good.

This way of eating is addictive, and (literally) is a BIG reason our youth these days are developing big guts way before they reach their 40's. It's sad, really. Once you've become accustomed to eating this stuff, real food doesn't taste good to you.

Good news: you're on your way to healing from this addiction. You're getting healthier every day.

STEP 2: Limit Fast Food

Do you know someone who can't lose weight no matter what they do? Some people can actually go without eating for days and not lose weight. The reason their metabolism is so messed up is they've been consuming so many chemicals they have actually altered their brain, which screws up their metabolism. If you are one of those people, the first step you can take to recover normal metabolism (and yes, it IS possible to fix this) is to stop eating processed foods. Start eating real food: whole organic fruits and vegetables, a few nuts and seeds — and organic, humanely raised and slaughtered grass- fed meats, wild caught fish (not farm-raised) and organic dairy products. Raw dairy products are amazing, but you might have to do a little work to find them.

Don't expect yourself to get it perfectly in one step. Just up your game a notch at a time. Start with the fast foods. Try to eliminate them, except on rare occasions. And when you have to eat fast, pick a place that uses better ingredients. I have a taste once in a while for a fast food burger. I walk to Good Times because they advertise that their beef is free of hormones and antibiotics. I order a cheeseburger with everything, wrapped in lettuce (I'm gluten-free). I drink water and skip the fries. This satisfies my fast food craving, doesn't mess me up too much, and I'm only out four bucks!

It makes more sense to stop doing the bad stuff before you get all wound-up in the fancy, expensive, highest-quality foods like free range meats! If you get off the fast/processed food wagon, you'll be way healthier than you will if you continue doing all the wrong things while adding organic foods and supplements to your diet. And you'll save tons of money too.

You've heard Hollywood stars make remarks like, "I'm 80% raw." Your end goal in this chapter will to be 80% non-processed—or better!

The Best Meats

Once you get a handle on NOT doing the bad stuff, consider investing in your health and longevity by purchasing only organic, humanely raised meats. Mass-produced meats have a heck of a lot more junk in them than non-organic produce does, so if you can't go all organic, focus on going organic on the animal products first (think: food chain)! Even the non-hormone/antibiotic-containing meats that are not organic are better than the common stuff. If you have the money, do a little research to find a sustainable farmer/rancher in your area. Get to know the people who are raising and slaughtering the animals you are eating. There's energy in that which has an effect on your health. Yes, they cost a bunch more, but you are worth it. Do as much as you can without driving yourself crazy or broke.

I used to do all of it, but today, I don't have that much money, so I do what I can. That's life. I still refuse to drink tap water and carry my own

3-gallon glass jugs up and down 30 steps to my 3rd floor apartment, and consider it a blessing that it helps keep me strong at age 60+.

STEP 3: AVOID Unfermented SOY, the Anti-Food

In "The Whole Soy Story – The Dark Side of America's Favorite Health Food", Kaayla Daniel, PhD, CCN, offers some facts on soy that will make your hair stand on end.

First, soy is not real food. It contains several anti-nutrients that block your absorption of important minerals. The goitrogens in soy actually attack the thyroid gland. Daniel sites hundreds of studies that link soy to thyroid dysfunction, malnutrition, digestive problems, cognitive decline, reproductive disorders, and more!

The Westin Price Foundation sued the Illinois Department of Corrections for feeding inmates too much soy and causing a myriad of health problems. Check it out if you don't believe it: http://www.westonaprice.org/soy-alert/.

The only soy that is OK to eat is the soy that has been naturally fermented for two years or more. Natural (with time, not chemicals) fermentation is the only method that is effective in removing soy's anti-nutrients. They tried it and nothing worked. Heating won't do it. Processing won't do it. Chemicals won't do it. The only soy foods I know of that are safe to eat are miso, tamari, tempeh, and natto. I'm really sorry, but edamame is not fermented either. Because it is young soybean, edamame may not be as high in concentrations of anti-nutrients, but it still feels like an unlikely food to me. I used to eat tofu, dry-roasted soybeans, edamame and soy milk regularly when I was in my teens. Perhaps that's why I have low thyroid function today.

There is so much confusion over soy that it is really important to do a bit of research and find out what rings true for you. PLEASE NOTE: Make sure each time you read an opinion about soy—whether pro or con—that you find out who wrote it and what connection they have with the soy industry! I've found entire websites devoted to the benefits of soy—as well as slyly placed opinions—which are owned and operated by none other than the makers of soy products such as Soy Joy. I highly recommend Daniel's book because she is not being paid or prompted by the soy industry or its antagonists.

STEP 4: Cook More Often

When you eat out at most restaurants—even the better ones—you have to assume you're getting some stuff on your plate that isn't real food at all. I'm not suggesting you never allow yourself to eat out. But please consider cooking in more often.

The only way you can be sure you're eating real food is to prepare it yourself. I know most people don't think they have enough time to cook. You will eat better, feel more balanced, and develop a relationship with the natural world

–which has a wonderful way of de-stressing you—by preparing your own food more often. And it's not that difficult if you follow the steps in this chapter.

I often cook with no other seasonings than sea salt and pepper, and I eat incredibly delicious meals all the time. I also really enjoy cooking when I play some nice music and sip on a glass of red wine.

Grab your meat or fish and whatever veggies you have in the fridge. Melt some coconut oil or ghee, and sauté whatever veggies you're in the mood for; broil, grill, poach or bake your fish or meat and you're done. Easier still, throw your meat on top of a pile of spring greens dressed with olive oil, balsamic vinegar, salt and pepper. Voilà!

It's so easy. You don't need recipes. You just need to have some fun experimenting with combinations of veggies, play with some herbs like cilantro and basil, goof around with different ways to cook your meats and fish and you'll find meals are really easy and fulfilling!

Try sprinkling Sea Seasonings' Gomisio on your veggies. It adds a delicious sesame flavor, and the seaweed in it feeds your thyroid gland. (Remember: your healthy thyroid contributes to faster metabolism!) I love steamed veggies topped with some melted butter or ghee and then sprinkled with gomisio.

I don't often use recipes. I just have fun and sometimes come up with astoundingly tasty dishes. Here are few of my favorites. Some were purely accidental.

* * *

Sue's Beef Basil Stir-fry

Start with a pound of good, hormone antibiotic-free sirloin. Rub with ghee, balsamic vinegar, sea salt, and cracked pepper. Marinate 1 or more hours in the fridge.

Put a little coconut oil or ghee in your fry pan and heat the pan pretty hot (but not so hot your oil smokes), then sear the sirloin on both sides. Remove from pan. The center of the steak should be raw.

Deglaze pan with a little water. Add onions and coconut oil as needed while you stir-fry the onions, then broccoli, and then yellow squash, then lots of shitake mushrooms. Add sea salt, cracked pepper and tamari while cooking. Meanwhile, slice the sirloin in thin strips. When veggies are just done, throw 3-4 handfuls of fresh basil leaves and wilt them. Then add the sirloin strips in, stirring around just until the steak is warm and done to your liking.

Serve with sliced tomatoes or beets for extra color.

Nan's Chicken Picatta

Buy a couple of good-looking chicken breasts, butterfly and pound them to ¼" thickness.

Sear the chicken in a fry pan with coconut oil or ghee. While searing, squeeze a fresh lemon over the breasts, add sea salt and pepper, and spoon a bunch of capers over them.

Remove chicken from pan when done (careful not to overcook; I like the middles slightly pink); leave capers in the pan. Pour in white wine and deglaze the pan, adding a chunk of butter too. Taste and see if you want more lemon, salt etc.

Pour the sauce with capers over the breasts and eat with tomatoes and fresh basil, drizzled with olive oil and a touch of balsamic vinegar.

Accidental Pork with Snap Peas and Mango

Dry your pork well so it will brown nicely. Brown natural pork chunks in coconut oil or

172

ghee with Celtic sea salt and plenty of cracked pepper and remove from pan. Deglaze pan with a little water, add a few cloves of garlic*, then put 2 or 3 handfuls of snap peas into the water. Grind some salt in.

Stir over medium-high heat just until snap peas start to steam. You don't need to cook them much at all. Then add chopped mango, fresh or frozen, stirring and cooking the snap peas more as the mixture gets syrupy. Add a pinch of cayenne pepper.

Finally add pork chunks back in, with two handfuls of fresh chopped cilantro. Heat through on high, without overcooking the pork. WOW!

Garnish plate with sliced avocado.

*I recently made this without garlic. It was still incredible! You can also substitute green beans for the snap peas.

* * *

Remember:

All you need for a meal is some quality protein, vegetables, and healthy fats. How you mix those together can be a creative, fun and delicious experience. Live a little! Unlock your creativity in the kitchen by sipping a glass of red wine and playing come great music while you cook.

…and don't forget to light some candles.

STEP 5: Plan Ahead

A well-stocked kitchen will save you more time and stress than you can imagine. All you need to do is get yourself organized and develop a few routines. You will find that preparing your own food can be really easy, quick and yummy.

Start here:

Personalize, then make two copies of the STAPLES list below and keep one in the glove compartment of your car and one on your fridge.

SUE'S STAPLES LIST

Protein Sources
Fish (wild-caught, not farm raised); Meats (no hormones or antibiotics); Low fat hard cheeses; Eggs (cage free); Sausages (less fat than protein per serving); Cottage cheese; Whey or egg white protein powder (unflavored, unsweetened) NEVER SOY!

Probiotics
Kefir (full fat, plain); Yogurt (full fat, plain); Probiotic supplement, Probiotic drinks, Live sauerkraut.

Produce
All fresh and frozen veggies and fruits I like EXCEPT for corn, potatoes, bananas, and mangos. Basil, Cilantro. Wild rice and grains only if they are gluten free. (Remember to soak them overnight to remove phytates); An occasional

red potato for a treat with steak.
Nuts and Seeds
Flax and/or chia seeds; Almonds, Walnuts, Cashews, Pecans, Pine nuts, Macadamias, Sunflower and pumpkin seeds.
Superfoods
Bee pollen (local, bulk); Fresh turmeric root, Fresh ginger root, Reishi mushroom powder with cracked spores, Coffee (Hey it's a superfood to me!—organic, fair trade); Various herbs for making teas and infusions; Herbal tea bags; Seaweeds (dulse, wakame, kelp hijiki).
Condiments
Celtic gray sea salt; Black pepper; Herbs and spices I like (non-irradiated and organic), Salsa, Hot sauce, Organic raw cider vinegar, Balsamic vinegar; Gomisio; Wheat-free tamari

176

Fats for Eating Raw
Olive oil (extra virgin, cold pressed); Butter (organic); Coconut oil (raw, organic)
Fats for Cooking
Coconut oil (organic, raw); Butter; Ghee
Miscellaneous
Water (first choice: fill my tanks at the spring; second choice: fill my tanks at the reverse osmosis machine); Don't drink tap water if you can help it. Don't buy water in disposable plastic bottles that will end in the landfill.
Sweeteners and Treats
Chocolate (dark, high quality with no corn sweeteners or mystery chemicals); Stevia (whole leaf, with no added dextrose or other sugars); Raw black honey; Grade B dark maple syrup; Boulder potato chips cooked in coconut oil; (an "occasional" treat, and

always eaten with lots of low-fat cottage cheese for protein); Red wines.

Give yourself some attainable goals and break them down:

- I will cook three meals at home this week
- I will carry a water bottle with me and drink it instead of sweet drinks
- I will cook this weekend and freeze some in portions for the workweek
- This week I'll keep a baggie of protein snacks with me at all times.

...things like that.

Try starting a habit of doing the week's grocery shopping on your day off.

Keep a working shopping list on the fridge and add to it during the week. Even better: download the free Evernote app, which syncs across all your electronic devices, and keep your list in there. Jot down what you need every time something pops into your head. On the weekend, check your cupboards against your staples list, and then grab your completed shopping list and go.

Become a Master of Freeze

Consider cooking on the weekends and freezing portions. I like to make a big pot of soup or stew and jar it up in pint-sized wide mouth mason jars and freeze them. It's a nice feeling to know I don't have to worry about what I'll eat for my next meal. If I can't come up with anything better, I've always got some soup! And storing food in glass is better than plastic. NOTE: Leave an inch of space at the top so the jars don't break when the food expands in the freezer.

I have developed the habit of taking something from the freezer (a jar of soup or stew, and maybe some fish or meat) and putting it in the fridge to thaw before I go to bed. Then tomorrow's meals are just about taken care of.

Always have your freezer loaded with fish, meat and frozen fruit. You'll never get stuck without good food available! I cut my meats and fish into serving sizes and re-wrap them individually, then put them in a large freezer bag before freezing.

Wrap up your food tight - like a chef. When my mom was a nanny for a chef's children, she noticed how meticulously he would tightly wrap pieces of things like veggies, fruits and cheese in plastic wrap before stashing in the fridge. When you take care about keeping the air out of your food packages, you will be amazed at how much fresher it stays—for longer.

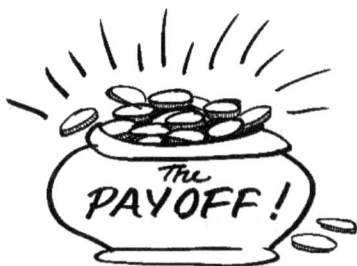

The PAYOFF!

If you're on track with this program, you really deserve your best body ever! You're:

- Steering clear of unhealthy chemicals in foods
- Gradually turning away from fast food meals
- Avoiding soy that's not fermented
- Having fun in the kitchen – cooking!
- Becoming more organized about meals

Your payoff? Your brain chemistry has balanced, which is causing your metabolism to normalize. You're not having to starve yourself anymore to avoid gaining weight. You're feeling clcancr inside and out—and more grounded and calm. Chances are, you're sleeping better. Your thyroid function is improving, which is increasing your metabolic rate. Cooking is making you happier, and you're feeling more connected with the natural world. If you're cooking with your mate, your relationship is improving! And you're less stressed-out because of your newfound super-organized habits.

If that's not enough, Chapter 6 will give you some assistive nutritional supplements that can speed your healing process along!

Resources – Chapter 4

Pringle, Peter. Food, Inc.: Mendel to Monsanto-- The Promises and Perils of the Biotech Harvest. New York, NY: Simon & Schuster, 2003.

Daniel, Kaayla T., PhD, CCN. The Whole Soy Story: The Dark Side of America's Favorite Health Food. Washington, DC: New Trends Publishing, Inc., 2005

Schlosser, Eric. Fast Food Nation: The Dark Side of the All-American Meal. New York, NY: Houghton Mifflin Co., 2001.

Westin Price Foundation:
http://www.westonaprice.org/soy-alert/

Chapter 5:

The Skinny on Fats

You are really going to love this chapter, because I'm giving you the truth about fats.

* * *

TRUTH #1: FAT DOES NOT MAKE YOU FAT.

TRUTH #2: Saturated fat is good for you.

TRUTH #3: Polyunsaturated vegetable oils are NOT good for you.

* * *

I know this is difficult to believe. The medical profession has been telling you for decades to eat a low-fat diet and avoid saturated fats, including cholesterol. In their place, they've been telling you to eat poly-unsaturated vegetable oils—and to take statin medications to reduce your serum cholesterol. This misinformation is causing our national health to fail. (B-r-e-a-t-h-e.)

Are you old enough to remember the middle cover of Time Magazine from 1984? The image was hard to forget, and millions of people have gone without bacon and egg breakfasts for decades…and gotten fatter and sicker, and a little less satisfied along the way.

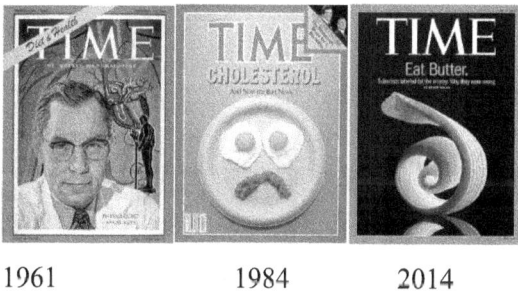

1961   1984   2014

The cholesterol and saturated fat myth was launched by a physiologist named Ancel Keys. Keys was so certain that he knew the reason for hcart disease that he created a study (The Seven Countries Study) that would prove his hypothesis. The bottom line is that Keys cherry-picked his data to confirm his hypothesis and the resulting devastation has manifested as our current epidemic of obesity, metabolic syndrome, Type 2 diabetes, heart disease, and cancer.

Back in 1961, Time ran Keys' photo on its cover with the "conclusions" he championed: that heart disease was caused by the consumption of saturated fats and cholesterol; and that people should not eat animal fats and instead should consume polyunsaturated fats. This was extremely unfortunate.

Time ran an apologetic cover article in 2014 titled, "EAT BUTTER: Scientists labeled fat the enemy. Why they were wrong." In case you missed it, you can Google the article, or "Ancel Keys" or "The Seven Countries Study" and be sure to read up on "benefits of saturated fats" and go wild. The Resources section after this chapter will get you started.

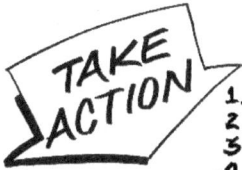

TAKE ACTION
1. EAT STABLE FATS
2. AVOID POLY-UNSATURATED OILS
3. EAT COCONUT OIL
4. TAKE AN OMEGA-3 SUPPLEMENT
5. DON'T HEAT OLIVE OIL
6. GET A LIPOPROTEIN PARTICLE PROFILE

STEP 1: Eat Stable Fats

Saturated fat is actually good for you because it is stable, which means it does not oxidize easily inside your body. Oxidation is bad, and causes a chain reaction of events in the body that lead to disease and aging. Saturated fat can be heated without becoming oxidized.

STEP 2: Don't Use Poly-unsaturated Oils

Polyunsaturated fats (vegetable oils) are unstable. They oxidize very rapidly and cause a series of physiologic events that cause free radical damage, including atherosclerosis.

By the way, reduced-fat foods can increase your chances of developing insulin resistance…and you know what that means. Reduced fat foods are usually processed to remove fat, which is often replaced with carbohydrates, sugar, and chemical fillers that are unhealthy. You know what that means too.

High LDL and triglyceride levels in your blood are not necessarily the result of eating animal fats. (Again, read: insulin response.)

The omega-6 fatty acids in poly-unsaturated oils are inflammatory and carcinogenic. This is not to say you shouldn't include some seeds and nuts in your diet. However, consuming nut, seed, and vegetable *oils* can throw off the balance of omega 3-6- and 9 fatty acids. Omega-6 oils are easy to get in your diet by eating a normal diet, whereas omega-3 fatty acids (fish oil, krill oil) are usually deficient in people's diets. Using saturated fats for cooking and mono-unsaturated fats raw (e.g. olive oil) would be a much better choice.

STEP 3: Eat Coconut Oil

The Fat That Helps You Lose Weight

…and protects your heart and liver too. We are talking about organic, unrefined, raw, coconut oil; not the refined, hydrogenated kind in packaged foods.

It seems a bit counter-intuitive that fat could actually aid in weight loss—but it's true.

Fats and oils are composed of fatty acids. You've heard fats classified by saturation (saturated vs. unsaturated). The second way to classify fats is based on the size or length of the fatty acid. There are short chain fatty acids (SCFA), medium chain fatty acids (MCFA), and long chain fatty acids (LCFA). Short chain fatty acids (SCFA) contain less than 6 carbon atoms, medium chain fatty acids (MCFA) have between 6-12 carbons, and long chain fatty acids (LCFA) have 14 or more carbon atoms. The reason fats are classified based on their length is because the size of the carbon chain influences the chemical and physical properties of the fatty acid—and how they are metabolized in your body.

About 98% of the dietary fat that humans consume from both plant and animal sources is composed of LCFA. Coconut oil is really unique because it is primarily composed of medium chain fatty acids (MCFA), with lauric acid constituting approximately 47% of coconut oil. Medium chain fatty acids (MCFA) are metabolized very differently from long chain fatty acids (LCFA). SCFAs are manufactured inside the gut, so we aren't concerned with them here.

Medium Chain Fatty Acid Benefits

Long chain fatty acids (LCFA) are not easily absorbed by the gastrointestinal tract and require a string of processes for metabolism. Eventually, they are stored as fat in the body, and provide some energy.

In contrast, the medium chain fatty acids found in coconut oil are absorbed by the gastrointestinal tract with ease. They are used directly by your body as ATP (the most basic form of energy) and are NOT stored in the body as fat! They actually ramp up your metabolism, causing you to burn more calories!

Coconut Oil Boosts Energy

Because the medium chain fatty acids found in coconut oil are easily and rapidly transported into the mitochondria, unlike long chain fatty acids, they are immediately used for energy, resulting in a burst of energy and thermogenesis (read: fat-burn), which subsequently increases metabolism. Yes, this boost in energy means you feel less lethargic, and it can help you feel less tired as you perform daily activities.

Several animal studies and clinical studies have proven that ingestion of coconut oil increases metabolism and decreases body fat both in animal studies performed on mice, and in humans. Medium chain fatty acids increase metabolism and promote the loss of fat while providing a burst of energy that increases physical endurance.

Evidence that Coconut Oil Decreases Body Fat

Numerous studies have shown that coconut oil clearly reduces body fat.

- When healthy men and women were administered either medium chain fatty acids or long chain fatty acids in addition to a diet similar in fat, protein, and carbohydrates for 12 weeks, the individuals who took medium chain fatty acids had significantly less body weight and, specifically, body fat (The Journal of Nutrition 131 (11): 2853-2859).

- Studies have also shown that medium chain fatty acids also increase the oxidation of long chain fatty acids that are already in your body, tucked away in your love handles (International Journal of Obesity and Related Metabolic Disorders: Journal of the International Association for the Study of Obesity 24 (9): 1158-1166).

- Similar to the animal studies, medium chain fatty acids also boost energy production by increasing thermogenesis, which speeds up metabolism in humans as well (Metabolism: Clinical and Experimental 38 (7): 641-648).

- In another study, people with high triglyceride levels were given medium chain fatty acids for eight weeks. In addition to decreasing body fat, their triglyceride levels were lowered by 14.5% (European Journal of Clinical Nutrition 63 (7): 879-886).

Coconut oil is a saturated fat. It is solid in temperatures up to 76 degrees, and liquid when warmer. Because saturated fats are stable, coconut oil is the ideal oil to cook with. It is also great to eat in its raw, unheated state. At times when I get cold due to thyroid malfunction or a Vata imbalance (that's an Ayurvedic term), I can eat a spoonful of coconut oil topped with Celtic Gray sea salt and within minutes my body is toasty warm. (Nibbling on dried dulse, the red seaweed, also works to warm me right up.)

To reap the benefits of coconut oil, you simply need to change the type of oil you use to cook with. If you're worried about the coconut taste, you can buy expeller pressed coconut oil, which has no coconut smell or flavor and is great for cooking (but it is not raw, so not as beneficial). Forget about the price. You're worth it. And you can save money by ordering it online.

STEP 4: Take an Omega-3 Supplement

Omega-3 Fatty Acids

Decades of research highlight the importance of the Omega-3 essential fatty acids eicosapentaenoic acid (EPA) and docosahexaenoic acid (DHA) for long-term health. These essential fatty acids offer unique support for inflammatory balance, cardiovascular function, and cognitive and emotional health. Getting adequate levels through dietary sources and/or supplementation is important.

Krill Oil:

Krill oil is my favorite source for Omega 3's. Although you can obtain Omega-3 fatty acids from a variety of sources (e.g. krill oil, fish oil, flax seed, and algae), they are not equal in potency or effectiveness. The vegetarian sources (except for algae-sourced) require an enzymatic process to yield the EPA and DHA; better sources are non-vegetarian. The anti-oxidant potency of krill oil has been found to be 48 times more potent than fish oil. Some manufacturers have figured out a way to give vegetarians the benefits of EPA and DHA from algae.

I choose to take one capsule of Krill oil daily for a month, and fish oil capsules on alternate months. Krill oil doesn't cause the "fish-burp" that fish oil does, and I like its additional strong antioxidant properties, which give it a longer shelf life too.

STEP 5: Don't Heat Olive Oil (Omega-9)

Olive oil contains mono-unsaturated fatty acids (omega-9) that are very good for you. However, the fatty acids in olive oil are not stable when heated, so reserve olive oil for salads, drizzling, or uncooked sauces. Macadamia nuts are another good source of mono-unsaturated fat. Use saturated fats (coconut oil, butter, and ghee) for cooking.

STEP 6: If you have high LDL cholesterol, ask your doctor for a Lipoprotein Particle Profile.

My naturopathic doctor had me take this test, which is offered by Spectracell Labs. The test did not cost very much at the time, and I was willing to do it because, although my HDL level is high and my triglycerides are low, I have a high LDL count. It turns out that my LDL molecules are mostly the large, buoyant kind, which aren't dangerous. Yay! See the link in the Resources for this chapter. Knowing that you are high in the Big LDL molecules may ease your mind and allow you to comfortably forgo dangerous cholesterol-lowering medications!

The FAT Bottom Line:

Ask yourself: "Why do I still believe the myths?" Then do what you feel is best, including possibly reading up on the information I've given you in the following Resource section. Try some of my suggestions and see how it feels.

I eat eggs every day and uncured bacon whenever the mood strikes. I eat red meat more often than white (I have blood type O…more on that in the next book)—and I eat poultry and fish regularly.

I only cook with saturated (stable) fats like coconut oil, butter, and ghee. I also eat coconut oil unheated. I eat olive oil freely, but try to never heat it. I don't consume polyunsaturated vegetable oils, except for those I get from eating a few raw nuts and seeds. I take fish and/or krill oil supplements, and I refuse to take statins, no matter what! That's *me. You need to decide what feels right and good for you.*

Almost forgot: If you love to go and eat out at fine restaurants, don't worry too much. Once your day-to-day habits are pretty good, you can feel totally free to eat whatever suits you when having that fun meal out. There's a balance to be enjoyed—between discipline and *total pleasure!*

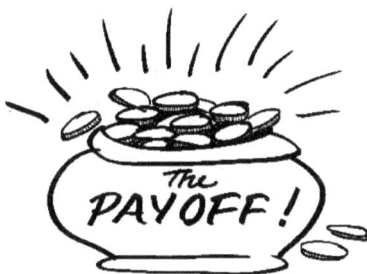

Following these steps:

- Cooking with stable (saturated) fats
- Forgoing polyunsaturated oils
- Eating raw coconut oil
- Taking an Omega-3 supplement
- Eating olive oil but not cooking with it
- Knowing the size of your LDL molecules

…will pay off significantly in your long-term health. First, you won't be unwittingly causing free-radical damage and inflammation, which lead to cardiovascular disease and aging processes. Your heart will be happier, and you'll cut your risk of cancer too. Your joints will be better lubricated, and you will reduce inflammation throughout your body systems. Free-radical damage, which is basically aging, will slow down. Your HDL cholesterol (the good kind) will go up and your LDL (the bad kind) will go down, as well as your triglycerides. If your LDL numbers are high still, you'll stop worrying about it if you do the Lipoprotein Particle Profile and find out that most of them are the large, buoyant kind.

Resources – Chapter 5

Spectracell Labs Lipoprotein Particle Profile
http://www.spectracell.com/clinicians/products/l
pp/

The Myth about Saturated Fats:

http://healthimpactnews.com/2014/time-
magazine-we-were-wrong-about-saturated-fats/

A brilliant young scientist, Chris Masterjohn,
debunks the cholesterol myth in this informative
interview:
(http://www.thelivinlowcarbshow.com/shownote
s/1326/chris-masterjohn-on-cholesterol-episode-
314/) Masterjohn is pursuing a PhD in
Nutritional Sciences with a concentration in
Biochemical and Molecular Nutrition at the
University of Connecticut. He has no ties to any
company or special interest group.

Read Chris Masterjohn's Daily Lipid blog to learn more about the virtues of unrefined coconut oil: http://blog.cholesterol-and-health.com/2010/06/coconut-not-only-protects-your-liver.html

Check out Stephan Guyenet's whole health blog: http://wholehealthsource.blogspot.com/2009/01/how-to-eat-grains.html. Guyenet received a B.S. in biochemistry from the University of Virginia in 2002, and a Ph.D. in neurobiology from the University of Washington in 2009. Professionally, he studies the neurobiology of body fat regulation. This blog is a free service to whoever wants to read it. It's supported by generous reader donations. Guyenet has no ties to any company or special interest group.

Coconut Oil:

http://nutritionreview.org/2013/04/medium-chain-triglycerides-mcts/

BOOKS

The Cholesterol Myths: Exposing the Fallacy
that Saturated Fat and Cholesterol Cause Heart
Disease, by Uffe Ravnskov, MD, PhD

Malignant Medical Myths: Why Medical
Treatment Causes 200,000 Deaths in the USA
each Year, and How to Protect Yourself, by Joel
M. Kauffman, Ph.D.

Lipitor: Thief of Memory, Statin Drugs and the
Misguided War on Cholesterol.
by Duane Graveline, M.D, M.P.H

www.thincs.org: The International Network of
Cholesterol Skeptics (THINCS) is a steadily
growing group of scientists, physicians, other
academicians and science writers from various
countries. Members of this group represent
different views about the causation of
atherosclerosis and cardiovascular disease,
some of them are in conflict with others, but
this is a normal part of science. "What we all

oppose is that animal fat and high cholesterol play a role. The aim with this website is to inform our colleagues and the public that this idea is not supported by scientific evidence; in fact, for many years a huge number of scientific studies have directly contradicted it." Visit www.thincs.org for a list of 88 medical doctors and scientists who are members.

Omega-3 Fatty Acids:

Omega-3 fatty acid supplements are typically sourced from fish oil, while plant-based omega-3 sources have historically contained alpha-linoleic acid (ALA), a precursor of EPA and DHA. Conversion of ALA from flaxseed and other vegetarian oils requires enzymatic conversion to EPA. A key enzyme in this process is delta-6-desaturase. The body's ability to covert ALA into EPA and DHA is highly variable from person to person. Newer manufacturing processes have recently begun to produce vegetarian, algae-sourced EPA and

DHA. Supplementation with plant-sourced EPA and DHA circumvents this enzymatic conversion step, providing vegetarians with the well-documented benefits of fish oils.

Krill oil comes from krill, which are small, shrimp like crustaceans that inhabit the cold ocean areas of the world, primarily the Antarctic and North Pacific Oceans. Krill make up the largest animal biomass on the planet.

Krill oil, like fish oil, contains both of the omega-3 fats, eicosapentanoic acid (EPA) and docosahexanoic acid (DHA), but hooked together in a different form. In fish oil, these omega-3 fatty acids are found in the triglyceride form, whereas in krill oil they are hooked up in a double chain phospholipid structure. The fats in our own cell walls are in the phospholipid form.

Attached to the EPA leg of the phospholipid is a molecule of astaxanthin, an extremely potent anti-oxidant. The phospholipid structure of the EPA and DHA in krill oil makes them much more absorbable and allows for easier entrance into the mitochondria and the cellular nucleus. In addition to EPA and DHA, krill oil contains a complex phospholipid profile including phosphatidylcholine, a potent source of stress-reducing choline.

Krill oil contains vitamin E, vitamin A, vitamin D and canthaxanthin, which is, like astaxanthin, a potent anti-oxidant. The anti-oxidant potency of krill oil is 48 times that of fish oil.

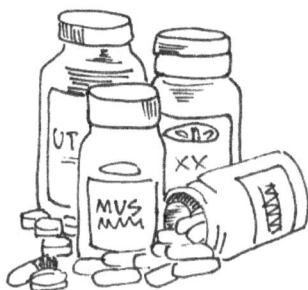

Chapter 6:

Supplements

Getting all tangled up in supplementation can be not only exhausting to your bank account; it can be dangerous to your health. Now that you've mastered chapters 1 through 5, you are absorbing an incredible array of nutrients. If we lived in an uncontaminated world, you wouldn't need to worry so much about supplements. That said, our world is not pristine, and there are a few supplements I recommend just about everybody *consider* taking. These are:

- Omega 3-fatty acid supplement

- Probiotic
- Folate in its naturally occurring, universally metabolized form, (L-5MTHF)
- Vitamin D3
- Magnesium
- Vitamin K2

Age matters. At the end of this chapter you'll find my suggestions for each age category: childhood, young adulthood; adults; and seniors. For those who have special genetic deficiencies or health issues, please consult your doctor.

When choosing from among the ridiculously diverse array of products and manufacturers, you really do—as much as you hate it—need to research the manufacturer before buying. Other than Primal Defense ULTRA, which is only made by one company, I purchase most of my supplements from a supplier that is science and evidence-based, and the company uses an extensive product testing program that involves verification of label claims, potency and purity by 3rd-party laboratories. I also like the fact that the company is socially responsible. You can access the supplements I use and recommend at SueRoseBlog.com.

Special Supplements:

PS—MEMORY PROBLEMS? FORGET ABOUT IT!

This amazing supplement, PS, or phosphatidylserine, supports age-associated memory decline as well as overall learning, recall and processing capacity in young adults and students. I noticed a big difference when I began taking it!

Individuals on cholinergic or acetylcholinesterase medications may require monitoring. Consult your physician.

7-Keto DHEA: WEIGHT LOSS HELPER!

When I was going to the fancy longevity doctors, DHEA was recommended across the board for assisting in weight loss and changing body composition toward more muscle and less fat. However, most DHEA supplements convert to testosterone or estrogen. (Girls, READ: WHISKERS) so I stopped taking it for years. I was thrilled to find 7-KETO DHEA, a safe and natural metabolite of DHEA. This form does not convert to either testosterone or estrogen, and has proven itself in studies to be several times more potent than DHEA in stimulating the thermogenic enzymes of the liver, promoting basal metabolism, and helping to increase the lean/adipose ratio. These actions safely support a leaner BMI (Body Mass Index) and healthy weight control.

Thyroid Support Complex

There is a reason the longevity doctors are prescribing thyroid hormones. The thyroid gland, like so many other parts of our bodies, tends to diminish as we age, making us feel lethargic, chilly, and fat. Not only that—most people have damaged their thyroid gland by eating soy and other food additives. An underactive thyroid means low energy, loss of hair, and weight gain! Take care of your thyroid gland and it will take care of you. In my next book we'll go through lots of ways you can stimulate your thyroid. For now, consider this wonderful supplement.

DIM

If you're a woman taking hormone replacement, whether HRT (hormone replacement therapy) or BHRT (bio identical hormone replacement therapy), DIM has been recommended by my doctors because it is protective against breast cancer due to high estrogen levels.

Ubiquinol (active Co-Q10)

Ubiquinol is the active antioxidant form of Co-Q10. Co-Q10 is well known for its ability to support cardiovascular health. It also enhances energy levels in every cell in the body, providing increased energy and exercise tolerance.

However, as we age, some people are not able to convert CoQ10 (ubiquinone) into its active form, ubiquinol. For this reason, if you're over 40, you have a better chance of responding to supplementation with ubiquinol. For those of you who are taking statins, this is a critical supplement because statins diminish the level of Co-Q10 in your body.

Across the Board Supplements:

Omega-3 Supplements (krill oil, fish oil, algae)

Most Omega-3 supplements will contain both omega-3 fatty acids, EPA and DHA; these will appear in a variety of proportions. The children's supplement is more focused on DHA because that's associated with mental and visual health and respiratory function. EPA is more associated with vascular health and healthy mood. In general, omega-3 fatty acids are well recognized for supporting cardiovascular function, emotional well being, and healthy skin and joints.

Krill oil has been shown to support some additional systems. It also assists in protection from the sun and environment, and contains the potent antioxidant astaxanthin, associated with eye health.

Because of a slight blood thinning effect, people on blood thinners need to check with their doctors before taking krill or fish oils.

Folate

Folic acid is a critical nutrient present in some foods. Scientists have discovered that some people have a genetic condition that prohibits folic acid assimilation. Fortunately, they've found a formulation of folate called L-5-MTHF that is directly metabolized by the body, even in people who can't process folic acid from food.

(I'm one of them, and I suspect my offspring are too.)

If you choose to take any of Pure Encapsulation's multiple supplements, most of them contain the L-5-MTHF form of folate – a wise choice. If you don't take any of their multiples such as Nutrient 950 with Vitamin K, you can take the L-5-MTHF alone, and it's not expensive.

I became acutely aware of the importance of folate when I learned of my inability to process folic acid and the association I made with my son, who was born with severe neurological conditions. Folic acid is a required supplement for pregnant women, because it is critical for nucleic acid and neurotransmitter synthesis, and cellular and neural protection. Studies have shown improvement in people with ADD/ADHD when treated with therapeutic doses of folate, which makes me wonder if some ADD/ADHD people share with me the same inability to metabolize folic acid?

Vitamin D3

Vitamin D levels have been shown to decline with age. It enhances your body's ability to absorb calcium, a very important benefit for bone health. It assists in cardiovascular functions, colon health and cellular health, including prostate and breast tissues. Vitamin D3 also contributes to healthy glucose metabolism. It's not expensive, and you can actually take a week's dose all at once, if you can remember to take it each week. I prefer a daily dosage. If you have your blood levels monitored, you can go higher—even up to 10,000 iu daily if your levels are low; but it is best to stay at or below 2000 iu daily if you do not monitor your blood levels.

Check with your doctor before adding Vitamin D3 to your program if you are taking the diuretics, digoxin or thiazide.

Longevity Nutrients:

Time and again, my medical and alternative physicians are WOWED when I show them the label of this supplement, which is designed for the "over 60 crowd"…even when they are selling a different line of supplements. This is a powerhouse of nutrients that supports cognitive, metabolic, cardiovascular, macular, and retinal protection. I started on this supplement at 50, because it's just *that good*.

Magnesium:

This is one of the most important minerals you can consume. I like to think of magnesium as a natural calming and relaxing agent. It soothes the mind. It allows your muscles to relax. Dr. Carolyn Dean, MD, ND, has written several books about this very important mineral and health.

According to Dean, 80% of everyone walking the planet is deficient in magnesium—and medications exacerbate our deficiencies by further leaching it out of our bodies. Fluoride

drains the magnesium from our bodies.
Supplementation with calcium also causes us to
lose magnesium. Ongoing magnesium
deficiency manifests in some pretty ugly ways:

- Numbness and tingling
- Muscle contractions and cramps
- Seizures
- Personality changes
- Abnormal heart rhythms.
- Coronary spasms

It is very important to pay attention to the ratio
of calcium to magnesium in any supplements
you take. Contrary to what was once thought,
the calcium to magnesium ratio should be 1:1 or
more on the *magnesium* side of the equation.
There are several forms of magnesium
(glycinate, chloride, lactate, carbonate, citrate,
oxide, hydroxide/sulfate, taurate and threonate),
and each has differing characteristics and rates
of absorption.

It's great to take Epsom salt baths too. Epsom salts (magnesium) are absorbed through the skin. Read Dr. Dean's books, *Death by Modern Medicine,* and *The Magnesium Miracle,* to learn lots more about the importance of magnesium supplementation and the dangers of calcium supplementation—and why she earned the Arrhythmia Alliance Outstanding Medical Contribution to Cardiac Rhythm Management Services Award in 2012.

Magnesium should be taken separately from bisphosphonate medications. Caution should be taken with concurrent use of potassium-sparing diuretics. It may also be contraindicated with certain antibiotics. Consult your physician for more information.

Avoid:

Calcium Supplements

I get upset when I hear of doctors prescribing calcium supplements. If you are lacking in calcium, you would do well to take Vitamin D3, magnesium, and Vitamin K2 rather than taking a calcium supplement. You have to take all of these because they work synergistically. When you do get calcium in a supplement, be sure you are getting equal or more magnesium to the calcium—because you will cause a deficiency in magnesium if you take more calcium than magnesium. Research suggests that simply adding Vitamin D can take care of calcium deficiencies. As you age, you really want to remain flexible, not brittle. Taking calcium supplements may not only cause you to die of a sudden heart attack—it also calcifies your body. Eat calcium-containing foods (e.g. dairy, broccoli, kale and collard and turnip greens; and herbal infusions like horsetail and oat straw) instead of calcium supplements.

Iron

Iron is neither man's best friend, nor a menopausal woman's.

Iron accumulates in the bodies of men and non-menstruating women. It never goes away. For this reason, I suggest people avoid multiple vitamin-mineral supplements that contain iron—unless they are young women or medically anemic. One famous doctor even recommends that men and menopausal women have phlebotomies in order to lower their serum ferritin levels. If you are a regular blood donor, you're doing yourself a huge favor. It turns out that, even though we need some iron, it is highly oxidative and damaging at elevated levels.

Afterword

I'm signing off for now, but there's lots more I would like to share with you. I'm thinking about remedies for when you're sick; simple devices you can buy that will enhance your vitality; digging deeper into herbs, Ayurvedic tricks, homeopathy and other alternative healing modalities; why barefoot is better; natural beauty secrets; advantages and pitfalls of hormone replacement therapies taken from my own rollercoaster experience; superfoods, and cooking for high vitality.

Cheers to you, *and* your best body—Go Out and CLAIM IT!

About the Author

Sue Rose lives and works in Colorado. She writes to help people connect with the natural world and become healthier and happier. Her favorite pastimes are hiking and snowshoeing in the mountains, wilderness camping, yoga, ballroom dancing, pickleball, writing, and learning to paint. Sue also runs Sue Rose Public Relations, a PR firm specializing in the architecture, engineering, and construction sector.

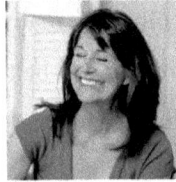

For additional copies of this book, visit Amazon.com or SueRoseBlog.com. Learn about Sue's lifescape and writing projects at SueRoseBlog.com.

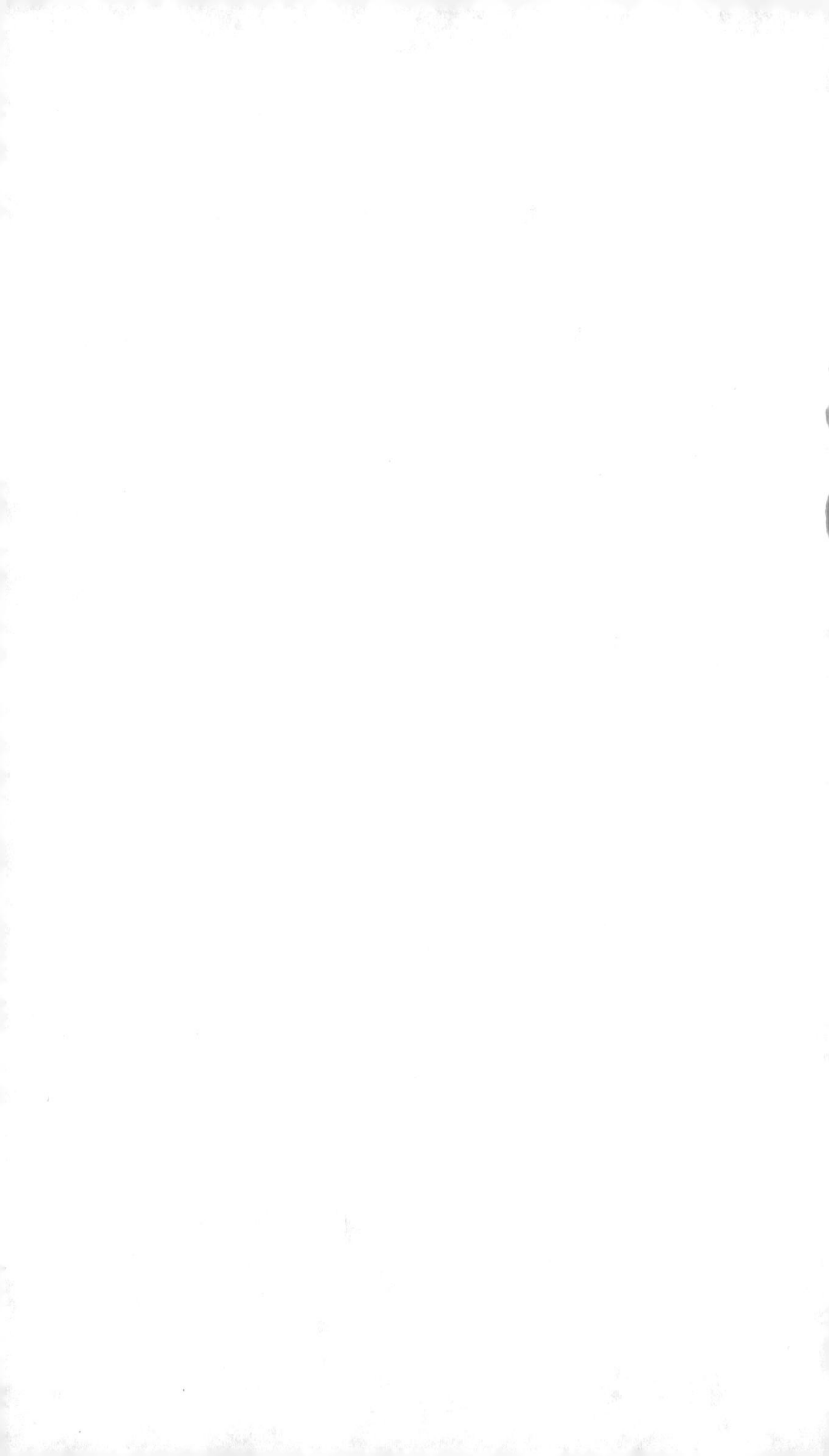